Clinical Standards Advisory Group

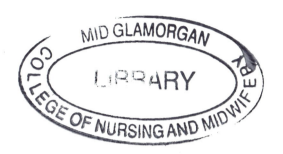
Urgent and Emergency Admissions to Hospital

The Report of a CSAG Committee
and the Government Response

Chairman Professor M Rosen, CBE
Study Director Dr R West

January 1995

London: HMSO

© Crown copyright 1995

Applications for reproduction should be made to HMSO
First published 1995

ISBN 0 11 321835 4

Preface

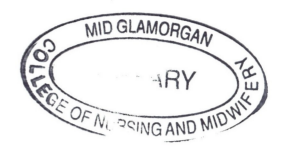

The Clinical Standards Advisory Group was set up in 1991, under Section 62 of the NHS and Community Care Act 1990, as an independent source of expert advice to the UK Health Ministers and to the NHS on standards of clinical care for, and access to and availability of services to, NHS patients.

The Group's members are nominated by the medical, nursing and dental Royal Colleges and their Faculties, and include the Chairmen of the Standing Medical, Nursing and Midwifery, and Dental Advisory Committees. Its investigations are carried out throughout the UK by members and co-opted experts, supported by research units under contract. Financial support is provided by the UK Health Departments, and the secretariat in based in the Department of Health, Wellington House, 133/155 Waterloo Road, London SE1 8UG.

This is the Group's fourth report. Its first three were on specialised services, diabetes and back pain; others will follow on maternity services, dental anaesthesia, schizophrenia, the elderly and elective surgery. All these remits were set by Ministers following advice from the Group.

Sir Gordon Higginson
Chairman, Clinical Standards Advisory Group

Contents

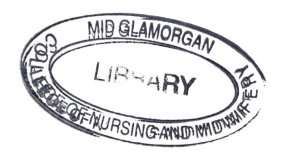

CSAG Report

Chapter 1

Introduction

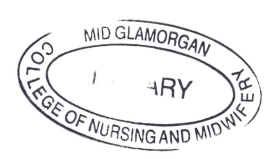

1.1   The subject of emergency services, including unplanned admissions, covers a wide range of health care activities both in primary care and in hospital. The standards of clinical care achieved will reflect access, availability, adequacy, quality, timeliness and effectiveness. Crucial questions about these can be answered by considering how patients reach hospital and how they are treated during the initial 24 hours.   Clinical management within the first 24 hours of an injury or acute illness may determine the outcome including early mortality, duration of hospital stay and residual disability which, in turn, may influence further or long-term demand for both hospital and primary care. The Clinical Standards Advisory Group (CSAG) considered it possible that, with increasingly detailed specification of standards in contracts for elective services, emergency services might receive less attention and even deteriorate unless they were examined and assessed. A study of current practice in a representative sample of acute general hospitals would be an important step in setting standards and in developing an audit cycle for monitoring and improving urgent/emergency medical care.

1.2   In January 1992 the UK Health Ministers asked CSAG to undertake such a study *to advise on standards of clinical care for patients admitted to hospital urgently or as emergencies. Your investigations will consider the time patients wait for diagnosis and treatment in the 24 hours after arrival at a hospital, and the factors influencing these times including events prior to arrival, in a representative sample of NHS hospitals. You will select several conditions for more detailed investigation, including if possible the effect on health outcomes of variations in the time patients wait.* CSAG established an Emergency Services Committee, composed of CSAG members and co-opted experts from relevant Royal Colleges (membership is listed at Appendix 6). The Committee designed a study in outline and selected a research group to develop the detail and undertake the study. The research team (listed at Appendix 7) worked closely with members of the Emergency Services Committee in this study of urgent and emergency admissions to hospital in a representative sample of districts in England, Wales, Scotland and Northern Ireland.

Chapter 2

Background

2.1 Setting standards

2.1.1   Setting standards for urgent or emergency admission to hospital and for the work of accident and emergency departments is complex and there are as yet no formal national standards or guidelines. Whilst a standards 'philosophy' underpins the "Working for Patients" White Paper (Department of Health, 1989) and the "Patients Charter" (Department of Health, 1991), the NHS reforms placed the main responsibility for setting standards with regions and districts. Some key national documents relevant to the development of standards in urgent and emergency admissions include the Royal College of Surgeons "Report on the management of patients with major injuries" (1988), the British Association for Accident & Emergency Medicine "Medical staffing in accident and emergency departments" (1991), the Department of Health "Welfare of children and young people in hospital" (1991), the National Audit Office "Report on accident and emergency departments in England" (1992) and the report of the Scottish Health Management Efficiency Group "Multidisciplinary group on accident and emergency services" (1992). However, much of the development of standards can be found only in unreferenced policy documents of regional or district health authorities (the 'grey literature'), written specifically for local use (for example Yorkshire Regional Health Authority's "Principles for emergency and urgent care in Yorkshire", 1992).

2.1.2   The "Patients Charter" was perhaps the most influential document on standards but, for urgent and emergency admission, the Charter set a specific national standard only for immediate assessment (or 'triage'). The Royal College of Surgeons report on trauma drew attention to the need for immediate availability of clinical skills in a variety of specialties. The National Audit Office report identified four key quality issues: medical staffing and supervision, timely support from other specialties, nurse staffing and management of workload. It also emphasised the importance of facilities for children, liaison with GPs, community health services and ambulance services and clinical audit, but only touched lightly on clinical issues.

2.1.3   Standards are increasingly being incorporated locally into purchasers' specifications for accident and emergency departments; for example, "patients should normally be treated, admitted to a ward or discharged within two hours of arriving". Some purchasers are attaching quality specifications to formal agreements with providers. Some agreements are including compliance (with 'charter standards') and applying a financial penalty (or 'bond') on a hospital that fails to achieve an agreed standard. In addition to the development of service specifications, an increasing number of diseases (e.g. asthma, cancer, cardiovascular disease, diabetes, accidents, mental illness, suicide, HIV and AIDS) are becoming subject to management by clinical protocols between GPs and consultants as a basis for agreed practice. The climate therefore is one in which standards of practice of urgent and emergency admission to hospital are being considered by both purchasers and providers (on a hospital to hospital basis) and agreements are being reached on what purchasers and, in turn, the public can expect from a particular hospital.

2.2   Numbers of urgent or emergency admissions

2.2.1   Statistics are available for discharges and deaths from NHS hospitals in England up to 1985 in the Hospital Inpatient Enquiry (HIPE). During the period 1979 to 1985 total deaths and discharges increased from 4,266,040 to 5,061,260, with immediate admissions comprising a nearly constant 50%. The number of day cases increased from 561,930 to 938,430 over the same period, but very few of these were immediate admissions. (OPCS 1981-1988, Milner PC et al 1988).

2.2.2   Hospital Episode Statistics (HES) for financial years from 1989-1990 record finished consultant episodes and include births, maternity and mental health admissions with acute admissions (OPCS 1993). Due to the break in continuity of published data and the new method of compiling statistics, direct comparison of the HES with the HIPE figures is difficult. However the HES figures indicate that the number of 'admissions' (1989-90:7.5 million, 1990-1:7.5m and 1991-2:7.8m) and use of day surgery (1.2m, 1.3m and 1.5m respectively) have both continued to increase and immediate 'admissions' comprised 58%, 57% and 56% respectively of all admissions (OPCS 1993, for the latter two financial years, OPCS unpublished.)

2.3   Need for urgent or emergency admission

Need for admission is most obviously determined by the seriousness of the patient's illness; when the patient's condition demands admission because, in the present state of knowledge, provision and practice of medical care, the most appropriate place for treatment or care is in hospital. The seriousness of a patient's illness may be described under three broad categories:

a)   critically ill: immediately life-threatening conditions, when timely and skilled treatment saves lives and reduces long term disability e.g. trauma care (Roy Coll Surg 1988, Champion MR et al 1990) thrombolysis in myocardial infarction (Mathey DG et al 1985, ISIS 2 1988). These patients all require admission.

b)   urgent/life threatening: patients with serious illnesses and injuries which have the potential to become immediately life-threatening if not treated quickly. Patients with haemorrhage, acute abdominal conditions and severe asthmatics fall into this category. Virtually all such patients will require admission.

c)   urgent/non-life threatening: patients with significant illnesses or injuries which may require admission. Examples include fractures of long bones, chest infections and various less severe abdominal complaints. Many will require admission.

d)   possibly urgent: there is a further group of patients for whom the reason for referral (or self-referral) is equivocal and the provisional diagnosis is uncertain. eg.

3

meningitis. Many of these patients justify admission for observation to clarify the diagnosis (although a proportion may be regarded subsequently as 'false alarms'.)

2.4 Variations in arrangements for urgent admission

There are wide variations in urgent admission arrangements from hospital to hospital across the country. Little is known as to whether these variations are attributable to differences in need, provision, priorities, standards or lack of knowledge of what is happening. The principal routes are outlined in below. The most frequent pattern for urgent referrals is that GPs (or other doctors) call specialist (or consultant) firms (direct to HO/SHO/registrar or via bed bureau) and admissions are direct to ward, to admissions unit or to accident and emergency and from there they are referred to specialist firms or are admitted to hospital beds. Some patients self-refer to accident and emergency (and then as above) or direct to specialist firms.

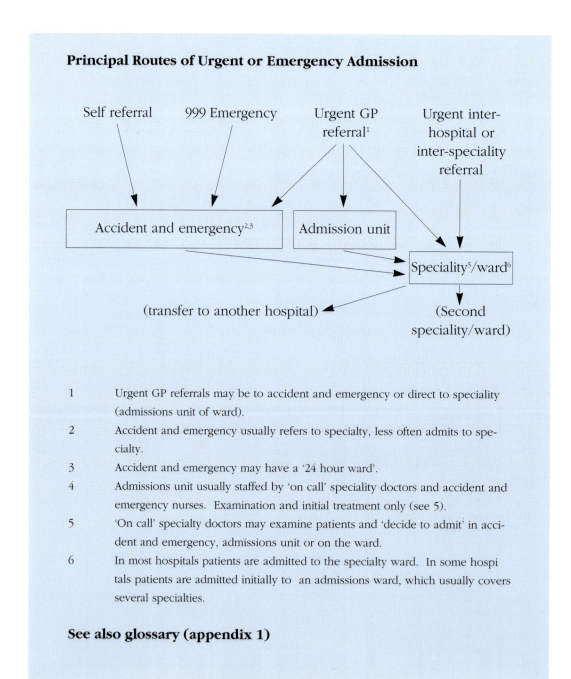

Principal Routes of Urgent or Emergency Admission

1 Urgent GP referrals may be to accident and emergency or direct to speciality (admissions unit of ward).

2 Accident and emergency usually refers to specialty, less often admits to specialty.

3 Accident and emergency may have a '24 hour ward'.

4 Admissions unit usually staffed by 'on call' speciality doctors and accident and emergency nurses. Examination and initial treatment only (see 5).

5 'On call' specialty doctors may examine patients and 'decide to admit' in accident and emergency, admissions unit or on the ward.

6 In most hospitals patients are admitted to the specialty ward. In some hospitals patients are admitted initially to an admissions ward, which usually covers several specialties.

See also glossary (appendix 1)

2.5   Management of resources

Effective management of scarce resources and best practice of acute care require good information on current activity, characteristics (or case mix) of urgent admissions, and on how urgent and emergency admissions are dealt with elsewhere.   In setting standards for urgent and emergency admissions there are a number of concepts and issues that need to be considered and balanced:

(i)   The 'trauma centre' concept of first line, top quality multi-specialist care for relatively rare events, in which highly qualified and highly skilled staff are on stand-by to attend rapidly when required.

(ii)   The issue of competing claims of urgent and elective patients for scarce resources, now used more efficiently, with little margin for the 'unexpected'. Efficiency is more easily obtained with an orderly and regular flow of elective patients, which may be at the expense of appropriate care of urgent patients.

(iii)   Closely associated is the issue of possible financial advantages to provider units in seeking and giving priority to contracts for elective work. This may lead to delaying discharges to protect beds for planned elective admissions - to make the specialty or hospital appear more efficient with elective admissions.

(iv)   A proportion of urgent referrals, often but not always less seriously ill patients, may be regarded as 'inappropriate'. These may tie up acute hospital beds and cause a burden on facilities for acute care unless strategies are developed to minimise such referrals and effect their early discharge (e.g. by use of observation wards).

(v)   Some self-referrals, described perhaps unfairly as 'inappropriate attenders', attend accident and emergency departments rather than consulting a general practitioner. Estimates of the numbers of such patients vary widely. While few require admission, they add to the workload of accident and emergency departments.

(vi)   The need for discharge planning or onward referral to the most appropriate long term care is widely acknowledged. Discharge management and liaison can greatly aid availability of acute beds for acute patients.

Chapter 3

Aims, objectives and study design

3.1   Aims and objectives

The study's principal aims were: to examine intervals between calling for urgent/emergency services, arrival at hospital, onset of definitive medical treatment and timing of key clinical events and to examine inter-district variation in these timings to see whether they cast light on the influence of district organization of urgent/emergency care on the promptness of medical treatment. The study included a follow-up review of clinical medical records designed to investigate associations between promptness and appropriateness of key clinical actions and 28 day outcome.

Specific objectives included:-

* Describing variety of provision, organisation and management of urgent and emergency admissions.

* Describing variety of urgent and emergency admission practice across the country.

* Measuring response time of ambulance services.

* Measuring time from arrival in hospital to onset of definitive management.

* Recording times of key clinical actions.

* Summarising key clinical actions.

* Examining the effect of management change on organisation of emergency services.

* Determining the effect of organization of emergency services on key clinical actions and their timing.

* Determining the influence of pre-hospital factors on key clinical actions and times.

* Estimating the influence of timing of key clinical actions on outcome.

* Estimating the influence of appropriateness of clinical actions on outcome.

3.2   Study design

The study was designed to observe all urgent or emergency admissions in a representative sample of 27 health districts (of the then 215 in England, Scotland, Wales and Northern Ireland), for 7 consecutive days in each chosen district. The districts were chosen as a stratified random sample to represent the country geographically, (compact 'urban' and dispersed 'rural') and in terms of health care organization (teaching and non-teaching, single admitting hospital and multiple admitting hospitals, concentration of specialties and dispersed specialties). The districts/hospitals studied are listed in Appendix 2.

3.2.1 Timing of key clinical actions

For seven consecutive days, 24 hours per day, teams of observers (doctors and nurses) monitored urgent and emergency admissions, timing the key clinical actions. Admissions to hospital for urgent or emergency patients may be through accident and emergency department, bed bureau or directly to wards, although activities may be concentrated in one area, and so in order to time events for patients being admitted, it was necessary to monitor all these entry points. Moreover, only a minority of patients attending accident and emergency departments are admitted to hospital and observers may not know whether or not a patient is being admitted until some medical assessment has been completed. Accordingly, the monitoring system needed to be capable of observing the significant key clinical decision/action and recording times for the subset of more seriously ill patients who were subsequently admitted without being bogged down in recording the bulk of accident and emergency activity. The monitoring system also needed to be capable of recording key clinical actions and the timing of significant events that occurred away from the emergency admissions area (i.e. in wards or in theatres).

3.2.2 Assessment of delays in admissions

Admissions procedures vary considerably in their complexity as patients pass between services, specialties, hospitals, wards or doctors and delays may occur for many reasons. An important feature of the observational study was to make an assessment as to whether a clinically significant delay occurred in any stage of delivery of the appropriate urgent or emergency care.

3.2.3 Assessment of outcome

The study reviewed after one month the clinical medical records of all patients admitted urgently or as emergencies during the study week to assess 28-day outcome. A brief summary of final diagnosis, duration of stay in hospital and (28 day) outcome was recorded.

3.2.4 Further analysis by condition

The principal diagnosis leading to admission and the principal final diagnosis were recorded so that specific conditions, e.g. orthopaedic trauma, abdominal trauma, ectopic pregnancy, head injury, asthma, stridor or croup in children, cardiac emergencies or gastro-intestinal bleeding, might be analysed later in more detail.

3.2.5 Hospital visits

Members of the CSAG Emergency Services Committee and the principal researchers visited all the hospitals to discuss with senior doctors, nurses and managers the local arrangements for urgent and emergency admissions so that the findings of the timing study could be put in context and suggestions considered for improving admissions procedures either locally or nationally.

Chapter 4   # Methods

4.1   Timing study

4.1.1   In each participating hospital, key times were observed for all patients admitted urgently or as emergencies, from when they entered the hospital to the time of definitive treatment or for the first 24 hours. Pre-hospital times were obtained from ambulance records for those patients who travelled by ambulance.

The following times were observed and recorded:

Pre-admission
- Time of first call (patient, GP or ambulance)*
- Time ambulance on scene *
- Time of arrival in hospital

Primary management
- Time doctor first attends
- Time of first clinical action
- Time of decision to refer to admitting team
- Time seen by admitting team

Definitive management
- Time of admission to ward/bed
- Time definitive management begins

from ambulance records

4.1.2   Times for each patient were recorded on a single form, starting with arrival in hospital. The form was so structured as to allow for the recording of times for a wide variety of urgent and emergency admission situations, together with diagnoses, investigations and treatments. Each form started with hospital and patient identification and subsequent sections covered 'Pre-admission', 'Admission', 'Primary management', 'Definitive management' and '28 day outcome'. The form is in Appendix 3.

4.1.3   The teams of doctor and nurses, gathering and recording the information, were generally based in the accident and emergency department and/or the emergency admissions unit of the participating hospitals, to allow first hand observations and timings of most key events. Observers also visited wards admitting patients, following admissions and recording times of key events personally and arranging for regular ward staff to enter the next relevant time, if personal observation by a member of the team was not possible. In the accident and emergency department forms were started for some patients who were not subsequently admitted, if it seemed that they might be, so as to avoid any omissions. In districts with a second hospital, to which urgent admissions were referred, the study team was enlarged. In districts with a second hospital, which received significant numbers of urgent admissions directly, a second study team was employed. The nurse coverage was concentrated on the busier times and in the busier units.

10

4.1.4   Urgent or emergency

Patients were classified in the following way:

- 999 Emergency - when patient, GP or proxy called an ambulance.

- GP Urgent - urgent admission requested by GP (or deputising service), whether to hospital bed bureau or direct to ward.

- Self-referral - (or walk in) first advice was arrival at accident and emergency.

- Other - Inter- or intra-hospital referral or transfer.

4.1.5   Recording of delays

Six stages where delays could occur were recorded:

- Ambulance bringing patient to hospital.

- Doctor attending patient on arrival.

- Onset of initial management.

- Admitting team seeing patient.

- Admission to definitive ward/specialty.

- Onset of definitive management.

As a general guide, delay was recorded if greater than one hour. However, there are clearly instances when a delay of less than one hour may be clinically important and judged significant by the observing team. These were therefore recorded. Guidance was given to nurse observers in a 10 page 'protocol', including representative clinical situations. When a delay was noted, the reason was recorded.

4.1.6   Pre-hospital (Ambulance) timings

Response time standards have been in use by the ambulance service for some years (14 minutes in urban areas and 19 minutes in rural areas). Ambulance staff therefore routinely log receipt of call, ambulance on scene and patient delivery in hospital. Many ambulance services have computerised records and were able to provide lists of patient deliveries classified by hospital, for 999 and urgent calls every 24 hours. These data were merged into the hospital timing record on a daily basis. For those ambulance services unable to provide 24 hour patient delivery listings, times were asked directly of the ambulanceman as each patient was delivered in accident and emergency/admissions unit. It was not a primary purpose of the study to measure ambulance response times, since these are routinely logged and target achievements recorded, but for completeness these times were linked to the hospital 'response times' for each patient. For GP admissions the study nurses recorded the timing of the call to bed bureau or directly to houseman or registrar, where possible.

4.1.7   Primary management

This covers the initial assessment, whether in the accident and emergency department, admissions Unit (receiving station) or ward, if the patient is directly admitted. The time of arrival and grade of the first doctor to examine and/or treat the patient were recorded. If two or more doctors arrived at almost the same time, the grade of the more senior doctor was recorded.

Time to triage was not measured. Admission via accident and emergency departments is only one of the routes into hospital for urgent and emergency patients, so many patients included in this study would not pass through triage. Furthermore, most patients who are triaged are not admitted and hence are not included in this study. In practice triage for the more seriously ill patient is usually informal and takes place immediately.

The primary provisional diagnosis was recorded: in many cases that was an initial presenting symptom rather than a definitive diagnosis (for example, 'chest pain' rather than 'myocardial infarction'). All diagnoses were coded to the International Classification of Diseases, ninth revision (ICD9). Final diagnoses were also recorded (see 4.1.12), particularly when these differed from the initial presenting diagnosis (for example 'myocardial infarction' rather than 'chest pain').

The initial investigations were those that took place as part of the first doctor's assessment or within the first hour of the patient's arrival in hospital (accident and emergency department, admissions unit or ward). Investigation included X-rays, blood tests, ECGs, respiratory function and ultrasound. Usually several (three or more) investigations were noted and the three most relevant to the presenting provisional diagnosis were coded. Similarly initial treatment was that undertaken as part of the first doctor's assessment in the receiving area (accident and emergency department, admissions unit or ward) and before the patient was transferred to another area (ward or theatre) for definitive treatment. Initial treatment may have been life saving (e.g. cardio pulmonary resuscitation), pain relief (e.g. for fracture prior to manipulation) or early 'definitive' treatment (e.g. thrombolysis in suspected myocardial infarction or administration of nebulisers and steroids for acute asthma, see below), or observation or monitoring. (Thrombolysis after transfer to a CCU or medical or geriatric ward or administration of nebuliser after transfer to medical or respiratory diseases ward would have counted as 'definitive' treatment.) Up to three initial treatments were coded.

4.1.8 Onward referral

Patients first seen in Accident and Emergency by Accident and Emergency staff and for whom admission is deemed appropriate are usually referred to an admitting team. The study recorded the time of the decision to refer to the admitting team and the time when they saw the patient, (whether in Accident and Emergency before admission to the ward or on the ward after admission). Patients seen initially by a receiving team, whether in a dedicated Admissions Unit or in a ward (or in Accident and Emergency) would have only one time recorded, since the time seen by the admitting team would be the same as the first 'time seen by medical officer'. Delays and perceived reasons for delays in decision to refer and in examination by the admitting team were recorded.

4.1.9 Definitive management

The time the patient was admitted to a bed in a ward was recorded, together with the specialty, any important delay in admission and the reason for any delay. The time definitive management (or operation) commenced was recorded, together with the grade of doctor responsible. For some patients definitive management was the same as initial or primary management. While for some others 'definitive management' entailed a period of observation. Significant delay of commencement of definitive management and reason for any delay were recorded.

4.1.10 Multiple referral

In rare complicated cases when urgent treatment was required in more than one specialty (for example in general surgery for soft tissue injuries and in orthopaedic surgery for fractures) a new form could be initiated at the decision to refer to (second) admitting team/admission to (second) ward/specialty stage, thereby allowing timings of the second definitive treatment to be recorded. Rather more commonly further treatment (in a second specialty), although relevant to the condition which led to urgent admission, was not urgently needed and followed the first definitive treatment (in the first specialty). In such cases timeliness was not a priority and the further treatment was recorded at follow up (see 4.1.12 below).

4.1.11 Collation of data

After twenty four hours the front sheet of the form was photocopied on site by the lead nurse or (senior) registrar and posted to study centre. In a few instances, however, if the patient was still waiting for definitive treatment, such as hip operation, the form was delayed until the operation had taken place. Normally, treatment which did not begin within 24 hours was recorded in the 28 day follow-up.

4.1.12 28 day outcome

The original forms were retained on-site for completion of the 28 day follow-up for which one of the observer team, usually the lead nurse, took responsibility. Four weeks after the timing study medical records were reviewed for final diagnosis (particularly if different from initial diagnosis), any further significant clinical action relevant to the urgent admission (that was not recorded during the initial 24 hours), 'disposal' (discharge, transfer to convalescent hospital, transfer to another specialty/hospital, still in hospital, dead) and duration of stay. In most hospitals the medical records were 'flagged' with a small study label and medical records staff collected most records in one place in readiness for the follow-up. In several hospitals the computerised patient administration system (PAS) was available.

4.1.13 Sample

The 215 District Health Authorities (DHAs) in England and Wales or Area Health Boards in Scotland and Northern Ireland at that time were stratified according to 'urbanness' (metropolitan, mainly urban or mainly rural), population, number of acute hospitals and teaching or non-teaching. Twenty seven districts were selected randomly from within these strata with the further restriction that each region was represented by at least one and not more than two districts, with Scotland, Northern Ireland and Wales each counting as one 'region'. The characteristics of the 27 selected districts were compared with those of all 215 districts to ensure that they satisfactorily represented the diversity of acute hospitals within the country. The districts and hospitals are listed in Appendix 2.

4.1.14 Approval

The dividing line between audit and research is not clear-cut. It was considered that although nothing was to be 'done' to patients and nothing was even to be 'asked of' patients, observations were to be made of individual patients and patient-specific data were to be analysed in a manner not normal in acute hospital patient care. It was considered, therefore, wise to seek ethical approval. The study was presented first to and approval granted by a medical ethics committee in a 'third party' district, since the principal investigator was a member of the ethics committee of the University teaching district where the study was piloted (see 4.1.16 below). Ethical approval was subsequently sought in this University teaching district. Approval was also sought in each district or hospital trust (see 4.1.15 below). In two sub-districts, one directly managed unit and one trust, formal local ethical committee application was requested and ethical approval was formally granted. Ethics committees and others have seen the study as audit rather than as research, and as raising no ethical difficulties.

4.1.15 Approach

The Chairman of the CSAG Emergency Services Committee wrote to the Chief Executive of Districts with directly managed units (or equivalent in Scotland and Northern Ireland) or of Trusts providing the principal acute services in those districts where Trusts had been formed, and to the Chairman of the District Medical Committee (or its equivalent) in directly managed units or of the principal provider unit Trusts, as appropriate. These letters referred to the letter by Sir Gordon Higginson, which introduced the Clinical Standards Advisory Group to District and Trust Chairmen (Jan 1992) and in turn introduced the UK Study of Urgent or Emergency Admission to Hospital and asked if the study might include their District or Trust.

4.1.16 Pilot

The study was piloted in full, including approach and approval (see above) in a district with three principal acute hospitals admitting urgent patients. The practical detail of timing observations was developed in three stages. In the first stage observations and timings were by the principal investigator and two senior registrars through most of 18 hours (8.00 a.m. to midnight) in all three hospitals concurrently. The study was described very briefly to medical and nursing staff. On occasions a timing form was left in the accident and emergency department, urgent admissions unit or (partly completed) in a ward to see whether regular staff in post entered the next patient or the time of the next significant action. The study was found to be feasible, first-hand timings were practicable for nearly 90 percent of actions and proxy or estimated times could be obtained for most of the remainder. The original draft timing sheet was modified somewhat in light of the first pilot.

The second phase of the pilot was to train a team of nurses to undertake the study for a full 24 hours. A full team of three nurses working 8 hour shifts was timetabled for the hospital 'on take' with partial 'office hours' cover for the other two hospitals to match the scheduled 'on take' rota and the known daily flow of urgent and emergency admissions. The study methods were described in some detail to these nurses and each carried a brief half page 'authorisation'. Most activity was observed first hand by a study nurse or estimated by interpolation only minutes after the event by a study nurse doing her ward rounds, following up urgent arrivals who were progressing through the admissions procedure. Proxy timings were obtained by telephone or retrospectively from regular staff in 'secondary hospitals' during night hours. Minor revisions to the timing sheet were made to make it easier to follow for both study nurses and regular staff.

The third stage of the pilot was a repeat of Stage 2 with a 28 day follow-up of records of patients, admitted during the second pilot, superimposed to test the feasibility of obtaining the 28 day follow-up information from medical records. The study methodology was developed through these pilot stages between May and July 1992.

4.2   Monitoring team

4.2.1   Nurses

The monitoring team in each study hospital district comprised 5 to 10 experienced and trained nurses under the supervision of a visiting registrar or senior registrar in accident and emergency medicine. While the principal task may be seen as 'organisation and methods' ('O and M') or clerical, the environment in which most of the timing measurements were made and the source of the information from which data were abstracted, made it essential that the members of the monitoring team should be acceptable to the medical and nursing staff in the urgent/emergency admitting hospital, should know their working practices, should recognise what was going on and to be familiar with the study hospital.

Nurses were selected, nominated and seconded to the study by the local district or hospital trust, which was reimbursed for nursing time. In single hospital districts, where most urgent and emergency admissions were concentrated in one hospital (or 'single-site' hospitals), about 5 or 6 nurses, working on rota, covered timing through the study week and one nurse, working social hours, was sufficient to collate information from ambulance records for the 28 day follow-up. In larger hospitals, where urgent or emergency admissions came through several routes (or 'split-site' hospitals) larger teams were employed and in 'multi-site' hospitals, two full teams were employed.

These administrative arrangements were discussed beforehand with the Royal College of Nursing.

4.2.2   Registrars/Senior Registrars

Five registrars/senior registrars in accident and emergency medicine were appointed as team supervisors. They had knowledge and experience of urgent admission procedures, the ability to recognize what was happening to patients (and what should be happening), the 'seniority' to ask what was happening and, as 'third party' observers (rather than as seconded employees of the observed hospital), were less likely to have preconceptions about the hospital's 'problem areas'. Each covered 5-9 districts, hospitals or hospital trusts. They were based on a hospital for 8 or 9 days, where they trained teams of nurses, supervised observations and checked procedures before moving on to the next district or hospital. They were seconded by their regular employing authorities for periods of 6-12 weeks to join the urgent admissions study. These arrangements were discussed beforehand with the British Association for Accident and Emergency Medicine.

4.2.3 Co-ordination

Supervision of monitoring teams in 27 districts was co-ordinated by a small research team (in Cardiff) which timetabled study weeks in sample districts, arranged attachments of study nurses, laid the ground for liaison with medical and nursing staff, medical records and ambulance control, liaised with travelling registrars/senior registrars, co-ordinated 28 day follow-ups by lead nurses and collected completed observation forms for data processing and analysis.

4.3 Committee visits to hospitals

4.3.1 Each district/hospital was visited by a member of the CSAG Emergency Services Committee. The visits were intended to clarify the local context within which the timing study was conducted (for interpretation of timing data), to gain understanding of the variety of urgent admissions procedures in different hospitals (as background for writing the report), to obtain first hand views of doctors, nurses and managers on problems affecting urgent admission, to develop two-way dialogue between members of CSAG Emergency Services Committee and those involved with managing urgent admissions (with the long term objective of improving procedures locally and nationally).

4.3.2 These visits were scheduled to take place after the timing study but before the district/hospital had received draft findings of its own timings. The visits were undertaken by one or two members of the Committee, with or without the principal researcher. The visitor(s) usually met a senior manager (Chief Executive or his nominated deputy), a senior surgeon (Director of Surgery, Chairman of Division or a surgeon concerned with urgent admissions), a senior physician (Director of Medicine, Chairman of Division or a physician involved with urgent admissions), a senior nurse, the Medical Director of the Accident and Emergency Department (and possibly an Administrative Director and a nurse supervisor of that department). The selection was left to the General Manager/Chief Executive of the hospital to arrange or delegate and the members of the hospital staff who met the visitor varied somewhat from hospital to hospital depending on availability. The visit was usually organised around three sessions with 2 or 3 members of staff at a time and a visit to the accident and emergency department, urgent admissions unit and 24 hour admissions ward as appropriate and typically lasted 4-5 hours in all.

4.4 Reporting back

We intend to copy the principal findings of the timing study to each participating hospital when our report is published. We shall give both the 'anonomized' timings included in this report and the hospital's own timings in confidence, so that each hospital may see how it compares with with others in timings of urgent and emergency admissions.

Results

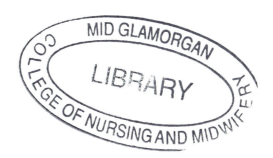

All 27 districts drawn in the representative random sample took part in the study and observations were made in the principal acute hospitals (directly managed or trusts) admitting urgent or emergency patients. In all 38 acute hospitals were included in the study. These have been classified as (i) 20 'single' hospitals, mostly self contained single site hospitals providing most 'district' specialties for acute care with little referral to another hospital and (ii) 10 multi-site hospitals or 'multiple hospital districts', where two or more hospitals share the principal 'district' specialties and/or where transfer from accident and emergency in one hospital to the relevant specialty in another is common. Six 'single' hospitals are situated in three districts, effectively providing the acute services for subdistricts within districts. The analysis includes 30 hospitals.

The timing study took place between September 1992 and March 1993 and the hospital visits by committee members took place between November 1992 and June 1993.

5.1   Timing study

Admission timings were obtained for 7757 patients. The number of patients observed in each 'hospital' (see above) averaged 258, range 85 to 419.

The key times are arrival to when doctor first attends (5.1.2), arrival to admission (5.1.4) and arrival to definitive clinical management (5.1.4). Results are summarized in sequence of occurrence; prehospital, doctor attends, first clinical action, admission and definitive clinical management.

Key to figures *The timing data are presented in a common style throughout the figures. These show the cumulative percentage of patients 'seen', 'admitted' etc. within the times shown '10,20,30,...120 minutes' etc. The line sweeping from 0% to 100% shows the 'grand means' of all hospitals in the study. The 'whiskers' show the range of hospital means (ie. the cumulative percentages recorded in individual hospitals) at several key times (eg. 30 minutes) and the 'ticks' on the 'whiskers' show the means for each participating hospital. When fewer than 30 'ticks' are shown on a 'whisker', two or more hospitals have recorded the same cumulative percentage at that point in time or some hospitals have recorded too few observations for the mean to be of any significance.*

5.1.1 Time from first call to arrival in hospital

5.1.1.1 Pre hospital times were obtained for 4123 patients; 1689 (84%) emergency 999 admissions, 2083 (54%) urgent GP referrals and 52 (25%) other referrals. Few pre-hospital times were obtained for self referrals (272, 18%), since for most their first contact with the service is arrival. 24 hour ambulance service logs were scrutinised and were found to correlate closely with direct entries on study timing proformas. Those patients without pre hospital timings were in most cases therefore those who did not use the ambulance service. Children in particular were brought in by car, even for emergencies. While not a main aim of this study, ambulance timings are summarized briefly, for completeness and for the bearing they have on timings within hospital.

5.1.1.2 For emergency 999 admissions by ambulance (figure 1a)

Thirty four percent of emergency admissions reached hospital (accident and emergency) within 30 minutes of the call being received by the ambulance service, but the variation was quite wide with as many as 72% and as few as 8% arriving within that time in the fastest and slowest districts respectively. These wide variations cannot be wholly attributable to population density or distance from scene to hospital.

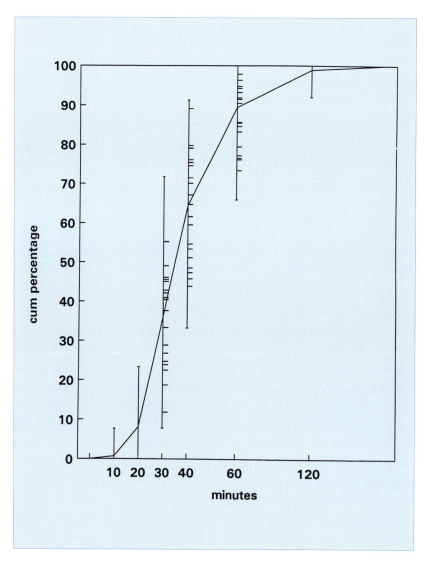

Figure 1a   Time from first call to arrival in hospital for emergency 999 admissions

5.1.1.3 For urgent GP referrals by ambulance (figure 1b)

The time between the call being received by the ambulance service and patients' arrival in hospital (accident and emergency, admissions unit or direct to ward) was considerably longer: 60% of patients reached hospital within one hour, again with quite wide variation between fastest (92%) and slowest (34%) districts. It should be appreciated that for many admissions these may not be emergencies; general practitioners often suggest or are asked to suggest a degree of urgency when booking an ambulance, for example "within 2 hours", and that these times should not be confused with ambulance 'response times'.

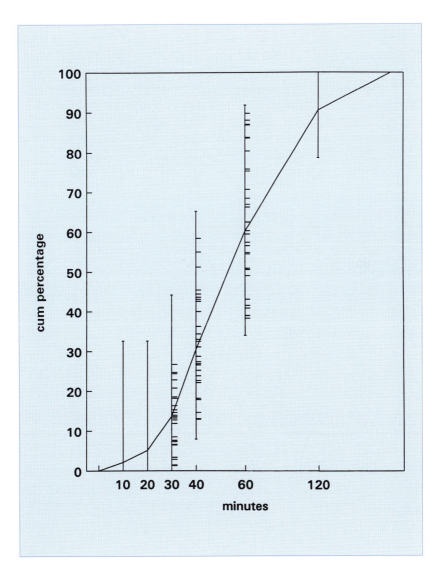

Figure 1b   Time from first call to arrival in hospital for urgent GP referrals

5.1.2 Time from arrival in hospital to first doctor attends

5.1.2.1 Inter-hospital variation (figure 2a)

59% of urgent or emergency patients were seen by a doctor within 30 minutes of arrival in hospital and 94% were seen within 2 hours. The median time from arrival to being seen was 23 minutes. However, there was significant variation between hospitals; the vertical bars in figure 2a show the range observed in 30 hospitals: 38% of patients were seen by a doctor within 30 minutes in the slowest hospital and 87% were seen in that time in the fastest hospital.

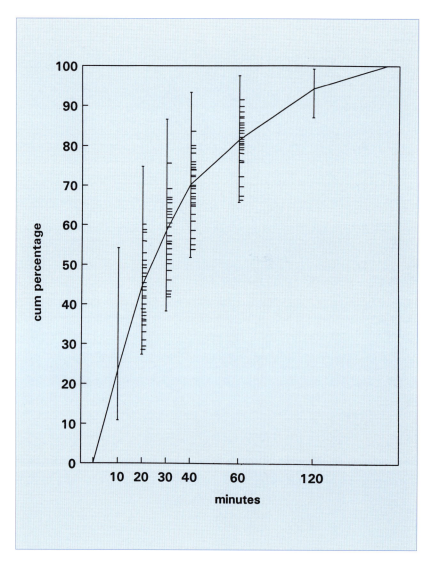

Figure 2a   Time of arrival in hospital to doctor attends (all patients)

5.1.2.2 By source of referral (figure 2b)

A difference was observed between emergency (999) referrals (28% of all urgent and emergency admissions) and urgent GP referrals (50% of all admissions): the former tend to be seen rather more quickly. Times for self-referrals (20% of all admissions) to be seen by a doctor were similar to those for emergency referrals, as might be expected since they mostly arrive at accident and emergency departments, and times for other referrals (2% of all admissions) are similar to those referred by GPs, as most are direct to ward. Inter-hospital variation in response times was evident within each class of referral (illustrated on the figure for 999 emergencies and GP referrals only at 30 minutes - for clarity) and inter-hospital variation far exceeds variation attributable to class of referral.

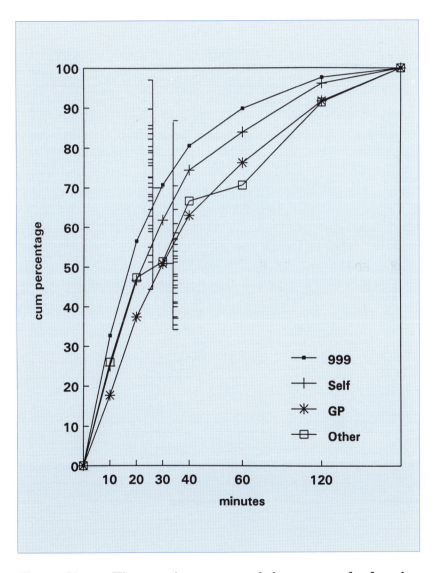

Figure 2b **Time to doctor attends by source of referral**

21

5.1.2.3 By day of week and by time of day (figure 2c)

Modest differences were observed in response time by day of week, with 56% of all urgent and emergency referrals being seen by a doctor within 30 minutes on Fridays and 66% on Sundays. Such variation may be expected since a higher proportion of admissions are 999 and via accident and emergency at weekends. There was rather more variation in response time by time of arrival (hour of day or night). While 72% were seen by a doctor within 30 minutes of arrival in hospital during the night (midnight till 9.00 a.m.), only 47% were seen within 30 minutes during the busiest hours in the early afternoon (midday till 3.00 p.m.). This reflects daily patterns of referral, with a higher proportion of admissions via 999 and accident and emergency by night, but it also suggests that staffing levels may not be sufficient to meet known and regular demand in the middle of the day. (Inter- hospital variation is shown only for arrivals between 3 pm and 6 pm, for clarity).

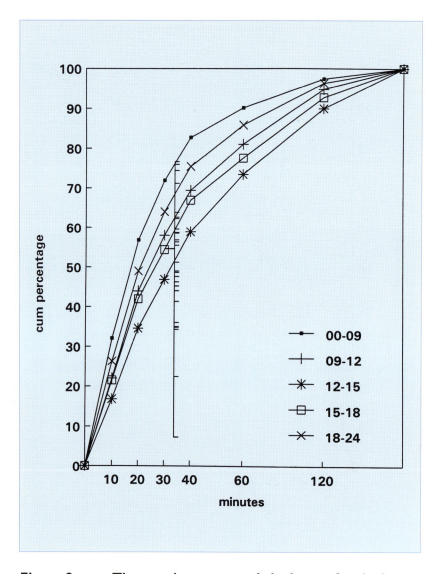

Figure 2c   Time to doctor attends by hour of arrival

5.1.2.4 By (grouped) diagnosis (figure 2d)

Patients referred for injuries (ICD 800-999) were generally seen more quickly (70% seen within 30 minutes) than patients presenting with respiratory conditions (ICD 460-514, 61% within 30 minutes) and those with circulatory conditions (ICD 390-459, 58% within 30 minutes). The differences between broad diagnostic groups reflect to some extent the observed variation by source of referral since most injuries arrive as 999 emergencies or self referrals at accident and emergency departments. Inter-hospital variation, shown in figure 2d for circulatory diseases seen within 30 minutes, is considerably wider than the variation between diagnostic groups.

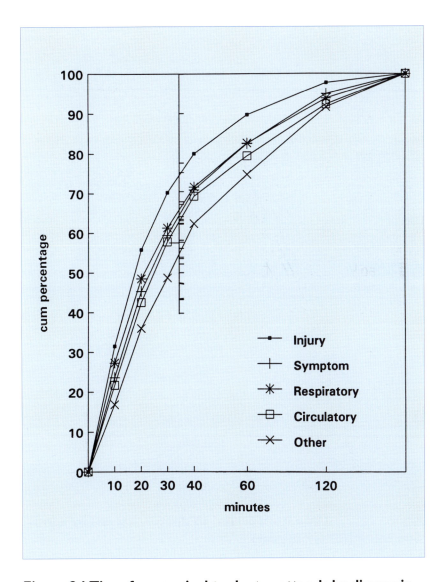

Figure 2d Time from arrival to doctor attends by diagnosis

5.1.2.5 By hospital admission route (figure 2e)

Hospitals were classified according to whether the majority of GP urgent admissions were direct to wards (specialties) or via Accident and Emergency departments. (Note, admissions in a hospital were not either wholly direct or wholly via Accident and Emergency. Gynaecology and paediatrics were often direct and orthopaedics often via accident and emergency). Patients were seen by a doctor rather sooner in those hospitals that employed the Accident and Emergency route for the majority of GP referrals, but differences were small and much less than 'random' inter-hospital differences.

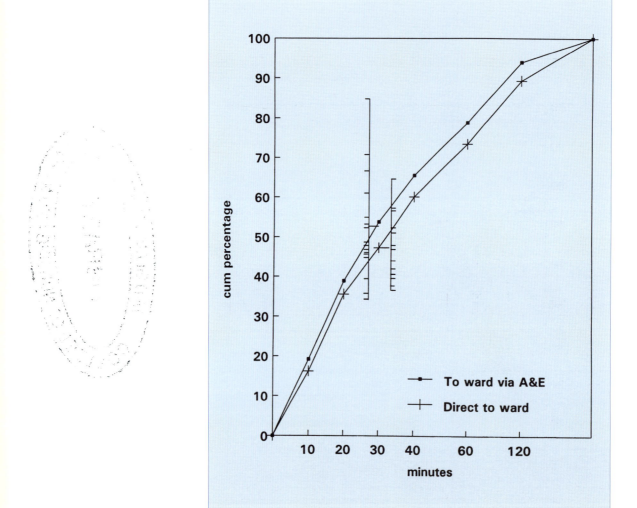

Figure 2e   Time from arrival to doctor attends by admission route (for GP urgent)

5.1.2.6. By hospital management

There were only modest differences in timings between 'single-site' hospitals and 'multi-site' hospitals (see glossary and section 5.1.4.4.), between directly managed units and trusts, between hospitals in metropolitan, urban or 'rural' districts or comparing hospitals that provided tertiary or 'regional' services (as well as typical 'district' services) and those that provided only typical 'district' services. However patients were not seen as quickly in hospitals in the 'South East' (hospitals in the four Thames health authority regions) as elsewhere in the country (see 5.1.4.6).

24

5.1.3 Time from arrival to initial clinical action

5.1.3.1 Inter-hospital variation (figure 3a)

Initial clinical action commenced within one hour for 69% of all urgent and emergency patients but again there was significant inter-hospital variation (range 43-91% at one hour). For an appreciable minority initial clinical action had not commenced within 2 hours of arrival (10%, range 1-29%) or within 4 hours of arrival (2%, range 0-5%).

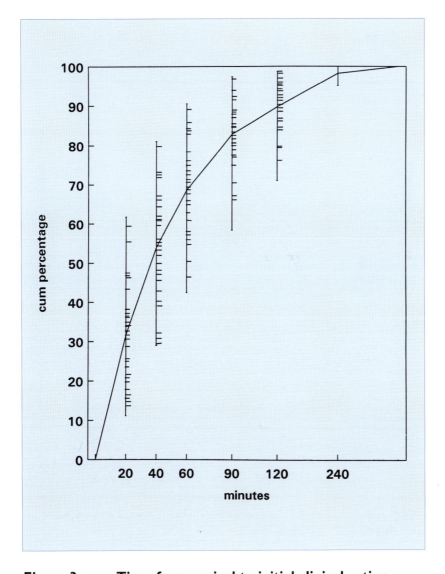

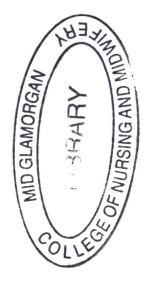

Figure 3a   **Time from arrival to initial clinical action**

5.1.3.2 By source of referral (figure 3b)

There was little difference between urgent (GP, self and other) and emergency (999) referral. At the median the difference amounted to barely 10 minutes. While emergency and self-referral patients tended to be seen more quickly (fig 2b) initial clinical action did not necessarily follow directly.

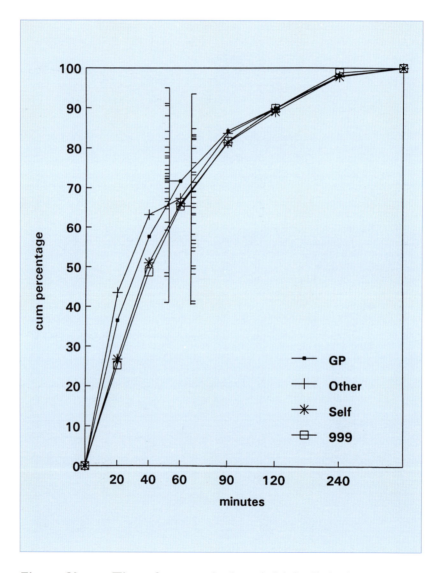

Figure 3b   Time from arrival to initial clinical action by source of referral

5.1.3.3 By (grouped) diagnosis (figure 3c)

Initial clinical action commenced rather sooner after arrival in hospital for those with respiratory symptoms than for those with injuries; at the median the difference amounted to approximately 15 minutes. At this level of grouping, diagnosis had little effect on time when clinical action began. Although diagnosis at finer detail would be expected to influence these response times, 'case mix is unlikely to explain the wide inter-hospital variations observed (in fig 3a).

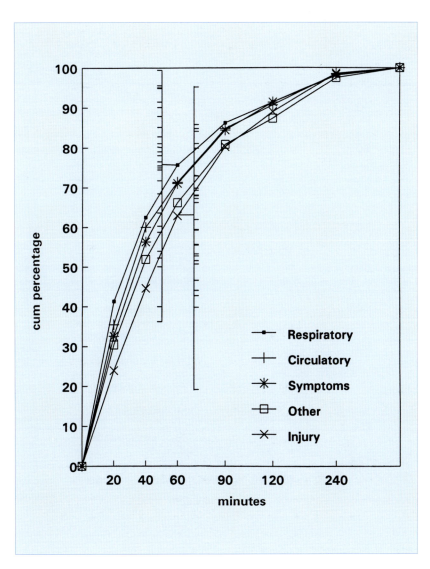

Figure 3c   Time from arrival to initial clinical action by diagnosis

5.1.3.4 By specialty (figure 3d)

Initial clinical action commenced earlier for patients admitted to paediatrics than for those admitted to orthopaedics: at the median the difference by specialty was about 25 minutes. While these interspecialty variations may be greater than variations by class of referral (fig 3b) or by grouped diagnosis (fig 3c), they remain smaller than the overall interhospital variation and, since the 'case mix' of urgent and emergency admissions is comparable between hospitals, much of the overall variation in response times remains unexplained.

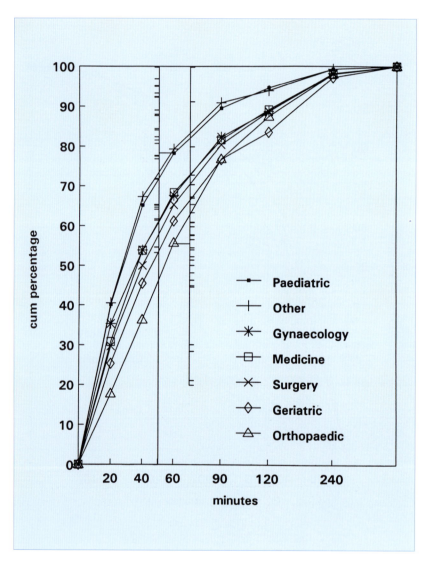

Figure 3c   Time from arrival to initial clinical action by speciality

5.1.3.5 By hospital management

'Single-site' hospitals had only a small lead over 'multi-site' hospitals in 999 emergency admissions, with no significant difference in GP urgent admissions. Timings were marginally faster in hospitals providing a 'district' service than those providing a tertiary or 'regional' service. These timings also tended to be slower in hospitals in the 'South East' than elsewhere in the country.

5.1.4   Time from arrival in hospital to admission to a bed in a ward

5.1.4.1 Inter-hospital variation (figure 4a)

About 39% of all urgent and emergency referrals were admitted to a bed within 1 hour but the inter-hospital variation was extreme (range 2% - 84%). After 4 hours a significant 13% remained unadmitted, again with a wide inter-hospital variation (0-66%). These wide variations owe more to the differences in route of admission (direct or via Accident and Emergency) than to delays in onset of clinical care (see relatively smaller variations in time to first clinical action in preceding section). Classifying hospitals (somewhat arbitrarily) as serving metropolitan, urban or 'rural' districts and comparing admission times showed that admissions were fastest in urban (median 91% admitted in 2 hours), followed by 'rural' (median 75%) and slowest in metropolitan hospitals (median 44%). The most striking feature of the

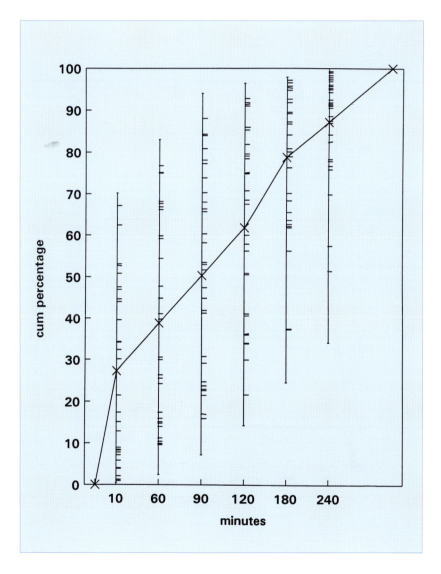

Figure 4a   Time from arrival to admission

inter-hospital variation was geographical: admission times were significantly slower in almost every hospital in the 'South East' than elsewhere (see 5.1.4.6 and figures 4f and 4g).

5.1.4.2 By source of referral (figure 4b)

Overall, 42% of GP urgent referrals were admitted directly (shown as within 10 minutes on figure). There was wide inter-hospital variation (range 0-85%), which reflects differences in hospital admission routes for GP referrals. Overall 69% of GP urgent referrals were admitted within two hours. This means that for those 58% of GP referrals not admitted directly, nearly half (47%) were admitted within two hours. For 999 emergency admissions also, 47% were admitted within 2 hours. For both GP referrals and 999 emergencies, extremely wide inter-hospital variations were observed; 20-99% and 10-100% respectively admitted within two hours.

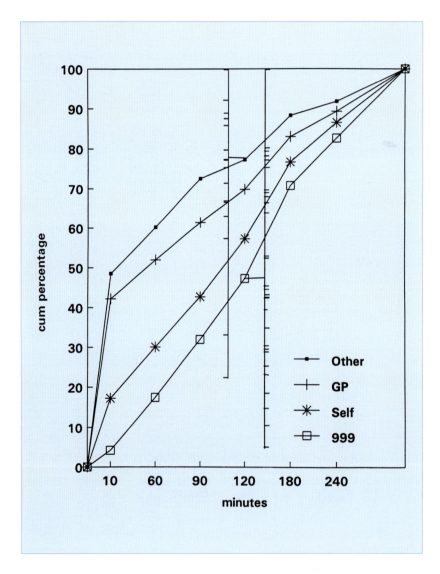

Figure 4b   Time from arrival to admission by source of referral

5.1.4.3 By specialty (figure 4c)

A very large variation between specialty was observed: 51% of urgent or emergency referrals to gynaecology were admitted directly (shown as within 10 minutes in figure range 0%-92%) and half (51%) of the remainder were admitted within two hours. 37% of urgent referrals to paediatrics are admitted directly and 65% of those not admitted directly were admitted within two hours. Only 41% of urgent referrals to orthopaedics reached a ward in two hours (range 0% to 100%).

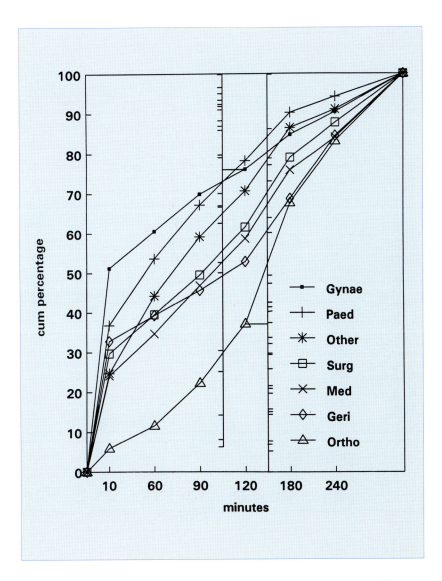

Figure 4c   Time from arrival to admission by speciality

5.1.4.4 For 'single' or 'multiple-site' hospitals (figure 4d)

No hospital was wholly self-contained (see glossary). Nevertheless, hospitals were classified into two broad classes: 'single-site' hospitals (20 in 17 districts) and 'multi-site' hospitals (10).

Admission times were rather shorter in 'multi-site' hospitals than in 'single-site' hospitals, with 53% and 43% respectively of 999 emergencies admitted within two hours and with 75% and 65% respectively of GP urgent referrals admitted within two hours.

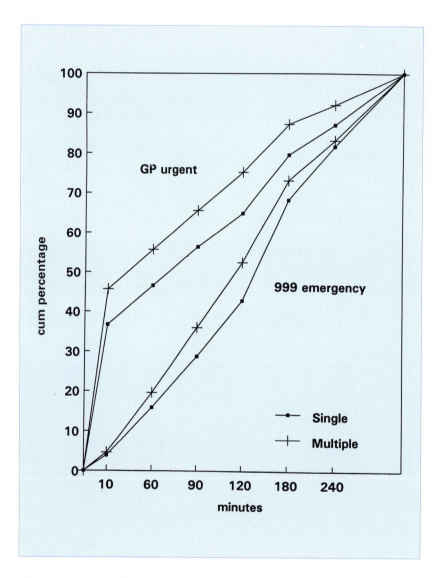

Figure 4d   Time from arrival to admission for single or multiple site hospitals

5.1.4.6 'South East' compared with the rest of UK (figures 4f and 4g)

Since admission times for GP urgent referrals depend on admission policy (straight to ward or via Accident and Emergency), the geographical variations in admission times are shown separately for 999 emergencies (figure 4f) and GP urgent referrals (figure 4g). Both show that hospitals in the 'South East' (the four Thames health authority regions) recorded significantly slower admission times than hospitals elsewhere in the country. Differences remained if the 'South East' were defined to include the four Thames health authority regions and the three regions bordering Greater London.

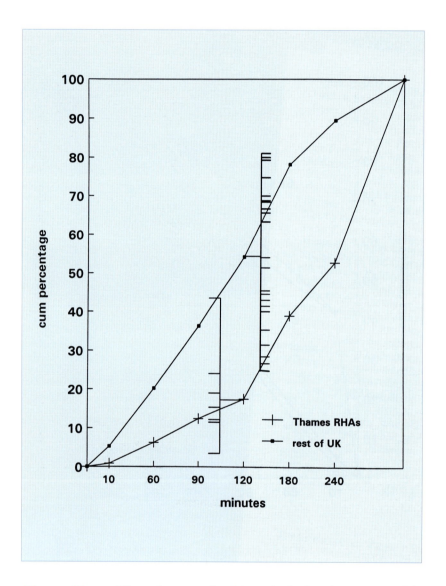

Figure 4f   Time from arrival to admission by geographical location for emergency 999 admissions

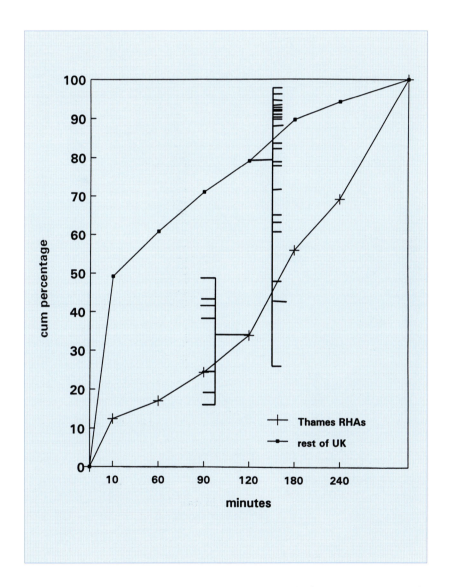

Figure 4g   Time from arrival to admission by geographical location for urgent GP referrals

5.1.5   Time from arrival to definitive management

5.1.5.1 Inter-hospital variation (figure 5a)

The median time from arrival in hospital to the start of definitive management was a little over 2 hours but the variation between hospitals in the proportion of patients whose definitive management commenced within 2 hours was wide: from 10% to 85%. Variations as wide as this cannot readily be explained by variation in class of referral, specialty, case mix or time of day etc, since most hospitals in the study include a comparable mix of urgent and emergency admissions and as the following figures show there was rather less relative variation in these times than in other key times (see previous sections).

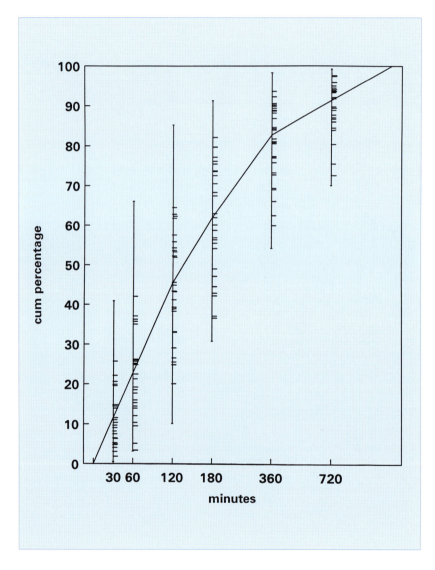

Figure 5a   Time from arrival to definitive management by hospital

36

5.1.5.2 By source of referral (figure 5b)

There was relatively little difference between urgent GP referrals and emergency 999 admissions. While previous timing comparisons (time to doctor attends, time to admission etc) showed different hospital admission procedures, for example that 999 emergencies are seen early (in accident and emergency) or that GP urgent patients are admitted directly in some hospitals, differences in admission procedures seem to have rather less impact on time to definitive management.

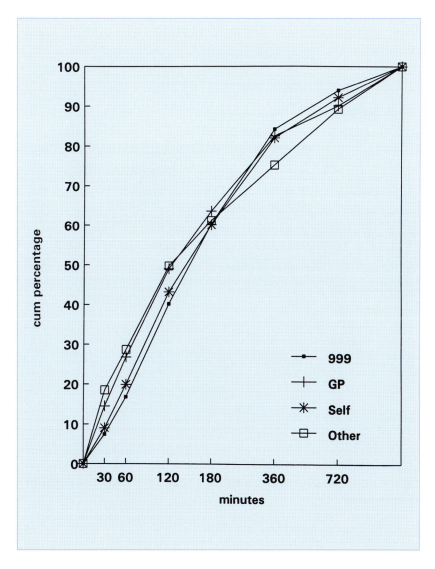

Figure 5b   Time from arrival to definitive management by source of referral

5.1.5.3 By specialty (figure 5c)

Definitive management commenced sooner after arrival in hospital for paediatrics patients (60% within 2 hours) and rather later for orthopaedic patients (27% within 2 hours).

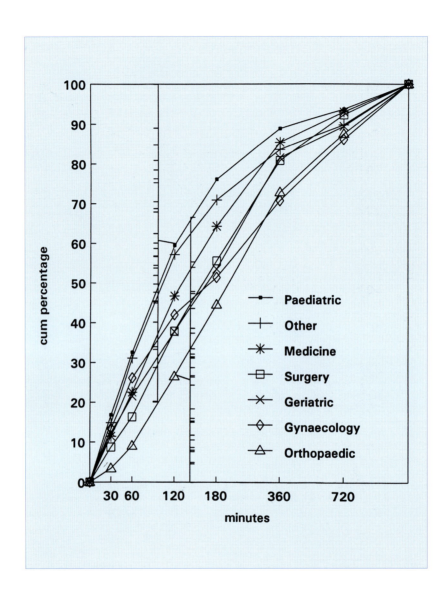

Figure 5c   Time from arrival to definitive management by speciality

5.1.5.4 By day of week and time of day

Definitive management commenced rather more promptly for patients who arrived on Sundays compared with those who arrived on weekdays and similarly for patients who arrived during night hours (6 pm - 9 am) compared with those who arrived during peak hours (9 am - 3 pm).

5.1.5.5 By (grouped) diagnosis (figure 5d)

Patients whose symptoms were indicative of respiratory disease received definitive treatment more promptly (55%, range 20% to 100% within 2 hours) and those with injuries rather less promptly (38%, range 6% to 86% within 2 hours). The inter-hospital variation cannot be attributed to difference in case mix.

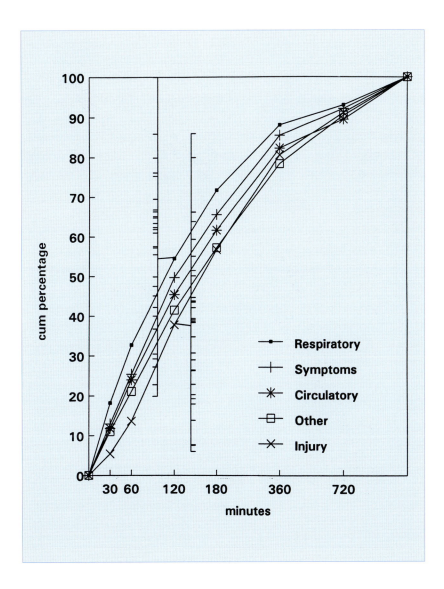

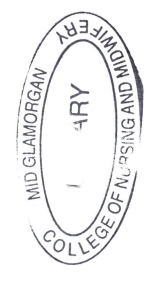

Figure 5d **Time from arrival to definitive management by diagnosis**

5.1.5.6 By hospital management

There were no significant differences between 'single-site' and 'multiple- site' hospitals. Definitive management commenced rather earlier in hospitals that provided a 'district' service than in those that provided a tertiary or 'regional' service and rather later in hospitals in the South East than elsehwere.

5.2 Delays - frequency and reasons (table 2a)

The observing teams recorded delays in doctor first attending, onset of initial clinical action, admission and definitive clinical management, with a guide threshold of 1 hour unless the patient's condition merited more urgent response. The frequency of recording of delays (percentage of patients) complements the more objective timing data and helps to identify where delays occur in the admission process in each study hospital. The frequencies of reported delays are summarised for the four key steps of admission and treatment of urgent and emergency patients in table 2a. The frequencies of perceived delays in each of the key steps of admission were closely correlated with the associated key timings; thus the hospital with the lowest percentage delay recorded in doctor first attending recorded (hospital a, top row in table 2a) was the hospital with the highest proportion of patients seen within 30 minutes (figure 2a). Table 2a shows some correlation between frequency of recorded delays by hospital in three key timings but little with 'definitive clinical management'. Thus in general hospitals that recorded few delays in 'doctor attending' also tended to record few delays in 'first clinical action' and 'admission'.

Table 2a   **Frequency of delays reported by the hospital: (percent of all urgent and emergency admissions)**

Percentage delay reported in

Hospital	Doctor first attending	initial clinical action	admission	definitive clinical management
a	4	8	20	4
b	4	5	6	7
c	5	2	14	11
d	5	5	5	5
e	6	7	8	2
f	7	3	13	17
g	7	11	6	12
h	8	16	24	7
i	8	11	5	9
j	8	3	5	5
k	9	9	19	4
l	10	4	15	23
m	10	5	9	18
n	11	8	7	11
o	11	6	22	6
p	12	5	9	12
q	12	10	8	2
r	12	7	8	4
s	13	18	15	10
t	13	9	7	13
u	14	4	5	7
v	15	11	22	14
w	16	16	33	1
x	16	3	13	15
y	16	9	7	12
z	16	6	16	9
aa	18	19	45	17
bb	27	15	62	6
cc	27	17	61	8
dd	28	27	63	17
all hospitals	12	9	17	9

* hospitals ranked (a-dd) according to the delay in doctor first attending (first column)

5.2.1 In doctor first attending (table 2b)

It was judged by the observing team that 12% of urgent and emergency admissions experienced delay in being seen by a doctor on arrival. There was wide inter-hospital variation (range 4 - 28%), just as in the timing data. Delays were twice as commonly recorded for GP urgent (15%) as for 999 emergency referrals (8%). This probably reflects the difference in working practices between wards (for direct admissions) and accident and emergency departments. Delays recorded for self-referrals and 'other' referrals were 10 and 12% respectively. There were also differences between specialties, with delays recorded more often for geriatrics (20%) than for paediatrics (8%), and between broad diagnostic groups, ranging between 14% for patients with circulatory diseases and 7% for those with injuries. While such differences may be understandable, they cannot be used to explain the main inter-hospital variation (table 2a).

The principal reasons identified for delay in doctor attending are summarised in table 2b, for the study as a whole and for three individual hospitals including those with the fewest and most recorded delays. The most common reason given for delay was that the responsible doctor was attending another patient (82%), followed by the responsible doctor attending a more urgent patient (11%). This may relate to inadequate staffing levels or inappropriate allocation of time. The timings of a further 261 urgent or emergency admissions suggested that delays may have occurred (an hour or more elapsed between arrival in hospital and doctor attending), but delay was not reported by the observing teams. These numbers have been added to the bottom of table 2b for completeness.

Table 2b   Reasons for delay in doctor first attending

Reason for delay	Hospital			
	a	l	dd	all
	(fewest delays)	(median)	(most delays)	hospitals
	Number (percent)			
Doctor with more urgent patient	1 (11)	0	5 (11)	100 (11)
Doctor with another patient	6 (67)	20 (95)	38 (81)	753 (82)
Doctor in theatre	1 (11)	0	2 (4)	27 (3)
Doctor on break	1 (11)	0	0	21 (2)
No bed	0	0	2 (4)	14 (2)
Patient non-urgent	0	1 (5)	0	8 (1)
Delay reported	9 (4)	21 (12)	47 (28)	923 (12)
Possible delay - no reason given	0	6 (3)	4 (2)	261 (3)

5.2.2 In initial clinical action (table 2c)

Initial clinical action was deemed to have been delayed in 9% of urgent and emergency patients. The inter-hospital variation was very similar to that for delay in doctor first attending (range 2 - 27%). However, perceived delay in onset of treatment was more common among 999 emergency patients (14%) than among GP urgent referrals (6%), the opposite of perceived delays in doctor first attending. This reflects differences in working practices and expectations of speed of response in emergency patients compared with GP urgent referrals, i.e. early assessment of 999 emergencies in accident and emergency departments and action following soon after arrival of the medical officer for GP referrals direct to wards. There were variations in percentage delayed by specialty, ranging from 5% in paediatrics to 13% in orthopaedics, and in grouped diagnosis, ranging from 5% among patients with respiratory diseases to 13% among those with injuries.

The main reason given for delay in onset of first clinical action was "no doctor" (46%), followed by "awaiting transfer - to ward or theatre" (20%) and waiting for X-ray (14%). (see table 2c). A further 323 patients (4% of all urgent and emergency admissions) whose timing data suggested that over an hour elapsed have been added for completeness.

Table 2c   Reasons for delay in onset of initial clinical action

Reason for delay	Hospital			
	c	n	dd	all
	(fewest delays)	(median)	(most delays)	hospitals
		Number (percent)		
No doctor	1 (20)	14 (38)	27 (59)	317 (46)
Waiting for opinion	2 (40)	0 (0)	10 (22)	65 (9)
Waiting for X-ray	0	9 (24)	4 (9)	94 (14)
Awaiting test results	0	3 (8)	4 (9)	51 (7)
Awaiting transfers	1 (20)	6 (16)	0	136 (20)
Porters	1 (20)	5 (14)	0 (2)	31 (31)
Delay reported	5 (2)	37 (8)	47 (27)	923 (9)
Possible delay - no reason given	4 (2)	10 (2)	1 (1)	323 (4)

5.2.3 In admission (table 2d)

Delay was deemed to have occurred more often in admission: 17% in the study as a whole. Delay in admission was recorded more often for 999 emergency (19%) than for GP urgent (16%), self referrals (15%) and other referrals (12%). The inter-specialty variation was much as before, with delay recorded more often for geriatrics (23%) and orthopaedics (18%) than for paediatrics (8%) and gynaecology (13%). There was little variation between main diagnostic groups. The inter-hospital variation was very substantial. Several hospitals recorded nearly half of admissions delayed and three recorded more than half delayed.

Table 2d	Reasons for delay in admission			
Reason for delay	Hospital			
	u	f	dd	all
	(fewest delays)	(median)	(most delays)	hospitals
	Number (percent)			
No bed	2 (13)	15 (43)	71 (66)	557 (43)
No doctor	4 (27)	5 (14)	11 (10)	204 (16)
No theatre	0	0	0	21 (2)
No porters	1 (7)	8 (23)	0	154 (4)
Awaiting diagnostic test results	4 (27)	0	4 (4)	51 (4)
Awaiting X-ray results	2 (13)	3 (9)	13 (12)	136 (11)
Awaiting transfer	2 (13)	4 (11)	8 (7)	164 (13)
Delay reported	15 (4)	35 (13)	107 63)	1287 (17)
Possible delay - no reason given	6 (2)	19 (7)	11 (7)	570 (7)

The main reasons for delay in admission (summarised in table 2d) were no beds (43% of those deemed delayed) and no doctor (16%), no porters (12%) (mostly for transfers within hospital) and awaiting transfer (to another hospital), (13%). There was relatively little variation in reasons between sources of referral or specialty. A further 570 patients (7% of all) whose timing suggested possible delay have been added for completeness.

44

5.2.4 For definitive clinical management (table 2e)

The overall frequency of recording delay in onset of definitive management was 9% (table 2a). An explanation for the frequency of recorded delays in definitive clinical management being lower than for admission is likely to be that some 'definitive clinical management' was initiated with 'initial clinical action' or before 'admission'. However it should also be appreciated that delay can occur at several stages in the admission process and that, if a delay was identified and the reason for delay recorded for say 'doctor first attending' or for 'admission', there was little point in repeating the same delay and giving the same reason. Therefore, delays recorded at this stage were mostly 'new' delays. Inter-hospital variation was again wide; range 1-23%. Delays in onset of definitive clinical management varied little by source of referral: 999 emergency (9%), self referrals (9%) and GP urgent referrals (10%) and other (12%). The inter-specialty comparisons showed gynaecology with the highest frequency (16%) and paediatrics with the lowest (10%).

The main reasons for delay in onset of definitive clinical management are summarised in table 2e. Half of these delays were attributed to no doctor being available and a quarter to no theatre being available. While the timing data suggested possible delays for a further 385 patients (5% of all), it should be borne in mind that for several procedures 'operation on the next list' (ie. next day) would be regarded as best practice.

Table 2e   Reasons for delay in onset of definitive clinical management

Reason for delay	Hospital w (fewest delays)		z (median)		I (most delays)		all hospitals	
	Number (percent)							
Patient non-urgent	0		6	(22)	8	(18)	68	(10)
No doctor	0		14	(52)	20	(44)	356	(50)
No theatre	0		0		9	(20)	195	(27)
Awaiting results	2	(67)	5	(19)	3	(7)	55	(8)
X-ray results	1	(33)	2	(7)	5	(11)	28	(4)
No beds	0		0		0		16	(2)
Delay reported	3	(1)	27	(9)	45	(23)	718	(9)
Possible delay - no reason given	13	(4)	22	(8)	12	(6)	385	(5)

5.3   Outcome at 28 days

5.3.1   28 day outcome (or 'disposal') by hospital (table 3a)

Most patients (83%) were discharged home by the time of the 28 day follow up, 1% were discharged to convalescent homes, 4% were still inpatients (in the admitting specialty), 2% in other specialties and 4% in other (acute) hospitals. Four hundred and sixty two patients (6%) had died (table 3a).

Emergency 999 patients were more likely to be still in hospital (8%) or in another hospital (4%) and self-referrals were less likely to be still in hospital (4%) or in another hospital (3%). Analysis by specialty showed a higher proportion still in hospital in geriatrics (15%) and 98% of gynaecology patients discharged home.

There were also differences in 28 day mortality by source of admission (999 emergency 7%, self-referrals 2%, GP urgent referrals 8% and other urgent referrals 6%) and by specialty (range paediatrics <1% to geriatrics 18%).

Table 3a shows considerable variation between hospitals in 28 day outcome, with the proportion discharged home ranging from 71-90% and with deaths ranging from 2-10%. Part of the variation may be due to source of referral and case mix, but it should also be remembered that hospitals in the study included the full range of urgent and emergency admissions.

One significant association was found between promptness of action following arrival in hospital, as measured by the 'key times', and 28 day mortality. Those hospitals that admitted a high proportion of their urgent and emergency patients within two hours (figure 4a) tended to have fewer 28 day deaths. (r = -0.37, p = 0.04). Promptness in doctor first attending, first clinical action and definitive clinical management pointed in the same direction, but none was statistically significant (at p < 0.05). The association between promptness of admission and 28 day mortality was balanced by a corresponding inverse association with proportion discharged (discharged home and to convalescent hospital combined). There was no association between any of the key admission times and the proportion still in hospital at 28 days (still in patient, other speciality and other hospital combined).

5.3.2   Length of hospital stay (table 3b)

The duration of stay of those patients discharged home within one month (28 days) is summarised in table 3b. In total, 24% of urgent or emergency admissions were discharged the following day. As with 'key times' the inter-hospital variation was wide, ranging from 6 to 39% discharged the following day. In all 76% were discharged within one week, with rather less interhospital variation, 62-89%.

No significant associations were observed between the key admission times and average duration of stay of patients discharged home after 28 days, nor between key times and proportion discharged after only 1 day. Thus there were no indications that hospitals that were quick to admit were also quick to discharge.

Table 3a   28 day outcome by hospital percent of patients

Percentage of patients

Hospital	discharged home	convales home	still inpatient	other speciality	other hospital	dead
a	90	0	3	2	1	4
b	89	2	1	0	2	6
c	89	0	4	1	3	4
d	88	1	3	2	1	5
e	88	0	5	2	2	4
f	87	2	3	3	1	4
g	87	1	6	<1	1	6
h	87	3	1	4	4	2
i	86	0	3	1	6	4
j	86	1	3	0	1	9
k	86	0	5	<1	4	5
l	86	0	1	<1	3	10
m	85	<1	4	3	4	4
n	84	4	4	2	2	5
o	84	3	1	2	22	7
p	84	6	3	2	0	6
q	83	<1	6	1	3	8
r	82	0	4	1	7	6
s	82	0	8	1	2	8
t	82	<1	1	1	10	6
u	81	1	8	4	1	6
v	79	8	2	4	4	4
w	79	1	4	1	11	6
x	78	1	7	1	5	8
y	77	<1	8	3	1	10
z	77	2	2	5	5	8
aa	76	0	3	10	1	10
bb	75	2	4	3	6	9
cc	74	8	4	1	6	7
dd	73	2	5	1	9	8
all hospitals	83	1	4	2	4	6

* Hospitals ranked (a-dd) by percent discharged home

Table 3b   Length of hospital stay (of patients discharged home)

Discharge home: cumulative percentage

Hospital*	1 day	-2 days	-4 days	-7 days	-14 days
a	22	39	59	74	91
b	19	34	52	69	90
c	17	43	65	81	95
d	31	47	64	80	88
e	10	39	60	78	88
f	36	52	64	79	90
g	24	35	55	74	91
h	27	41	57	76	94
i	6	29	51	73	90
j	22	35	51	73	88
k	123	28	49	67	89
l	25	41	62	73	89
m	24	44	63	82	94
n	29	45	61	78	90
o	28	40	56	74	89
p	23	36	52	75	92
q	37	52	69	82	96
r	16	41	64	81	95
s	35	46	63	77	92
t	32	43	66	82	93
u	22	30	49	64	87
v	16	37	54	72	90
w	21	38	58	80	94
x	9	34	57	72	87
y	27	41	60	77	92
z	29	38	51	68	89
aa	19	31	49	62	87
bb	19	30	45	66	87
cc	39	53	76	89	97
dd	15	38	62	76	89
all hospitals	24	40	59	76	92

* Hospitals ranked as in Table 3a

5.4   Hospital provision - questionnaire

Participating hospitals were sent questionnaires requesting background information about facilities, staffing, administrative arrangements and procedures for admission of urgent and emergency patients and about arrangements for audit and quality assurance.

This section is based on replies received from participating hospitals in twenty-one of twenty-seven districts. Some data, e.g. on facilities and attendance were obtained from other sources eg. CMA medical data (CMA 1992).

5.4.1   Attendance and admission data

The average annual number of new accident and emergency department attendances was 48,000, range 20,000 to 92,000. Expressed as a percentage of the district population attendance averaged 22%; range 14% to 26%, with one outlier, 46%.

The average annual number of unplanned admissions, both via accident and emergency and direct to ward was 17,500; range 10,500 to 35,500.

5.4.2   Staffing in accident and emergency

Most hospitals had one whole time consultant in accident and emergency medicine, six (larger) hospitals had two and one had four consultants. However, three districts of those that returned completed questionnaires, had no consultant in accident and emergency medicine and the departments were directed part-time by consultants from other specialties. The total number of doctors in post in accident and emergency departments averaged 10.6, range 5 to 16 and the number of medical staff in post matched numbers in establishment quite closely in most hospitals. The number of new attendances per doctor averaged 4,900; range 3,300 to 6,300. Nurse staffing ranged from about 20 to 30 (with one exceptional 60) depending on size of accident and emergency department and in general numbers in post matched establishment fairly closely.

5.4.3   24 hour specialties

Half of the hospitals (13) had 24 hour duty teams for all main specialties and four had teams available for nearly all specialties, excluding for example urology. However, eight hospitals (32%) did not have 24 hour cover on site for several major specialties (e.g. trauma, cardiology), although cover might be available elsewhere in the district. Nearly all hospitals had both intensive therapy unit and coronary care unit on site, but for two hospitals these units were elsewhere in the district. Eight hospitals (32%) reported having a high dependency unit.

Ten (40%) hospitals were not tertiary or regional referral centres, four provided one or two 'regional' specialties and ten provided a range of 'regional' specialties.

5.4.4   Diagnostic services

The majority of hospitals reported that their diagnostic service departments were available 24 hours a day but four did not have the complete range of services. Twelve hospitals reported they had MLSOs on site or on call after hours and nine did not.

5.4.5   Transfer of patients to other hospitals

Transfer of patients to another site in the same district for at least one specialty was widely reported. Nine hospitals transferred only a few specialties e.g. ophthalmology or severe head injury. Twelve hospitals, transferred several specialties, normally regarded as 'district' specialties. Transfer was usually by ambulance and only occasionally by private transport or taxi. The majority of hospitals quoted transfer times of 10-30 minutes, but four gave transfer times of 1-3 hours.

5.4.6   Triage, nurse practitioner and trauma team

Some form of 'triage' has been adopted in all but three of the hospitals, although for several hospitals 'triage' was somewhat informal, without dedicated space and - because of the degree of nursing commitment needed - without a senior nurse being formally attached. to that duty, on account of the nursing commitment required (see hospital visit).

Only three hospitals reported having a nurse practitioner scheme in accident and emergency. Only five had a trauma team.

5.4.7   Audit or quality assurance

The majority of hospitals (19) reported that quality assurance procedures were in place and/or that they had adopted medical audit. However only eight hospitals reported audit of accident and emergency. One hospital provided a report of a timing study, comparable to this study, for accident and emergency attendances and admissions. Similarly only six hospitals reported audit of urgent admissions.

Most hospitals recorded the number of complaints received from emergency patients. They averaged 17 per annum (range 4 to 44), and most were about medical care (the predominant complaint in 8 hospitals), and waiting time (2 hospitals). In one hospital, most complaints were about staff attitude.

Ten hospitals (40%) reported the use of computerised records in the accident and emergency departments.

Many hospitals (64%) indicated that they had plans for change in accident and emergency department including, for example, 'appoint accident and emergency consultant', 'upgrade waiting area' or 'introduce nurse practitioners'. Only a few gave details of plans for change in urgent admissions, for example 'implementation of bed bureau' or 'appointment of a bed manager'.

5.5   Findings of hospital visits

There was variety in provision for and organisation of urgent and emergency admission between hospitals and many different practices were observed in and described by hospitals in the study sample. Perceived problems of urgent or emergency admissions were differently addressed and solutions differed to the extent that newly instituted remedies at one hospital may be the discontinued practices of another. The following outlines issues that arose commonly and suggestions that were commonly offered as possible or partial solutions.

5.5.1   Provision

5.5.1.1 Funding arrangements There was broad consensus among managers and clinicians through most of the country that the funding arrangements with block contracts for urgent admissions but more detailed contracts specifying quantity and quality for elective admissions tended to favour the latter. It is relatively easy for both purchasers and providers to determine whether specific contracts in elective services are fulfilled and the consequences of any shortfall tend to fall on the emergency services.

5.5.1.2 Beds and space Whilst in many hospitals studied the overall bed provision was regarded as adequate for the average needs of the population served (based on average demand), this did not preclude difficulties in finding beds when needed. Bed provision was often described as inadequate for occasions of high demand. This could be particularly inconvenient at night, when patients had to be moved from one ward to another to make way for new patients. Many hospitals also described inappropriate distribution between specialties. Many accident and emergency departments were too small (Department of Health 1988, National Audit Office 1992). Some, although physically quite spacious, were poorly designed so that patient areas were cramped.

5.5.1.3 Staffing Many hospitals described shortages among accident and emergency medical staff, particularly among consultants and senior training grades, which made provision of adequate 24 hour supervision very onerous on those in post. Most single-handed consultants lived very locally (or even 'on campus') and were called into the department on many nights throughout the year. A role was seen for general practitioners within the accident and emergency departments if this were regular and well-integrated, or possibly to cover particular functions like primary care surgeries (Dale J et al. 1991). However, it was felt that poorly organised GP cover on an ad hoc sessional basis was of little advantage to accident and emergency departments. Medical staff shortages in accident and emergency departments are recognised and there are proposals to increase consultant numbers in England by 72 within three years 1992-5 (National Audit Office 1992). Many hospitals reported that nurse staffing was insufficient to provide 24 hour emergency theatre cover.

5.5.1.4 Buildings and sites 'Split-site' or 'multi-site' hospitals, where significant numbers of seriously ill patients need to be transferred between sites were regularly described as causing difficulties for urgent and emergency admissions. 'Split-sites' tie up both nurse and doctor time accompanying patients between hospitals. Consultants, senior registrars and registrars regularly waste one hour daily travelling between hospitals and different parts of their jobs. Several hospitals, both 'split-site' and large 'pavilionised' sites, were of poorly integrated design with accident and emergency departments separated from the principal admitting specialties. Such arrangements are dangerous and to be deprecated (National Audit Office 1992). Accident and emergency staff need support of the medical staff in the specialties of medicine (including geriatrics), surgery, anaesthesia, intensive care, paediatrics, orthopaedics, gynaecology, psychiatry and access to 24 hour diagnostic services. The siting of any of these in a hospital different from the one in which the accident and emergency department is situated may delay admission and the management of emergencies in these specialties. Isolation of the accident and emergency department also weakens co-operation and understanding between the junior medical staff in this department and the principal admitting specialties.

5.5.2   Factors outside hospital, that affect urgent and emergency admissions

5.5.2.1 Population served Several external factors were described as affecting urgent and emergency admissions or leading to difficulties for these admissions, most of which are outside the direct control of hospital management but, nevertheless, need to be considered in planning to provide adequate services to meet local demands. Certain characteristics of the population served affect demands made on emergency services. Particularly relevant in this aspect are the homeless (or rootless), visitors both long-term and short-term, and commuters. In some districts there are also relatively large populations of overseas visitors, immigrants or refugees, many of whom have both language difficulties and cultural misunderstandings of use of the GP and accident and emergency services.

5.5.2.2 GP referrals Wide variations have been reported in GP referral rates and GP referral thresholds generally (Royal College of General Practitioners 1974). Hospitals described similar variations in use of both the urgent and the accident and emergency routes to hospital. Some practices were regarded as providing inadequate cover for their patients, not only by night but also by day. Such unavailability has led to 'unnecessary' or 'inappropriate' attendances in some accident and emergency departments and to a perceived need for a primary care function or 'GP service' within accident and emergency.

5.5.2.3 Ambulance service Several hospitals wished to comment on how the ambulance service can affect urgent and emergency admissions and how management of patients by ambulance men can impinge on the management of these patients after arrival in hospital. Three areas of concern were raised. Some hospitals reported ambulance authorities' strong emphasis on increasing efficiency by maximising 'on road time' and suggested that this leads to over-hurried decanting of patients in hospital and unprofessionally cutting the hand-over of care and of relevant patient information. A few hospitals expressed concern at possible delays arising from treatment on site before transport, although it was generally considered that interventions by 'paramedics' were beneficial. The third area of concern was in difficulties obtaining ambulances for inter-hospital transfers, particularly in 'split-site' hospitals, which had led to some hospitals running their own inter-hospital ambulances.

5.5.2.4 Social services and admissions The availability of social services and community care affects both admissions and discharges. Shortfall in community care (particularly for the mentally ill in the community) makes higher demands on emergency services and on emergency admissions. Furthermore, arrival with poor (or no) referral letter, because patients are not being referred by doctors knowledgeable of their condition but are self-referring or being brought in by laymen, delays

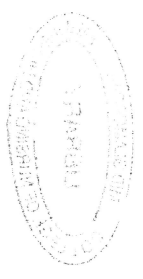

appropriate management. Many hospitals described the burden imposed by admissions for predominately 'social reasons', which may not be simply short-term overnight stays: initiating the cycle of medical investigation may lead to significant periods of hospitalisation. However, a few hospitals described good liaison arrangements, with 'on call' social workers and with Social Services' hostel beds, avoiding admitting patients for 'social reasons'.

5.5.2.5 Social Services and discharge The availability of social services and community care was referred to by all hospitals visited with respect to discharge and the effect discharge has on bed availability. 40% of urgent and emergency admissions are aged 65+ and many need continuing care after discharge (Jones DA et al 1993). While there should be an on-call social worker 24 hours per day to organise appropriate residential accommodation (eg. former part III) accommodation, many hospitals described difficulties in obtaining services and support at weekends and described difficulties in such things as obtaining social security payments for patients except on Thursdays. There was clearly an expressed need for good discharge liaison and good discharge planning (see 5.5.4.2), to ensure bed availability for further urgent and emergency admissions.

5.5.3 Management

5.5.3.1 Staff availability and rotas The committee visits found considerable variation between hospitals in organisational arrangements underpinning priority for urgent and emergency admissions, for example as to whether 'on take' teams were available 24 hours per day for all 'district general hospital' specialties and whether 'on take' teams in major admitting specialties were fully available for urgent admissions or had other duties (in outpatients or theatre) or duties in other hospitals on the same day. In some hospitals schedules and rotas seemed to be well organised and few delays were perceived to occur through doctors being tied up with other duties, while in others clashes of responsibility were reported relatively frequently with consequent delays in the early treatment of urgent admissions in some specialties. Some large departments (e.g. medicine) in the larger hospitals clearly enjoyed economies of scale.

5.5.3.2 Bed managers Good bed management was perceived to be the key to expeditious admission in all hospitals, although several did not have bed bureaus or had appointed bed managers only recently and only to cover 'office hours'. Bed managers should have seniority, authority and clear guidelines or protocols. One or two larger hospitals outlined detailed 'cascades' of specialties and wards that could be called upon to provide beds, when pressures built up in other specialties, that had been agreed previously by divisional directorates. Another aspect of bed management clearly identified by a few hospitals that has important consequences for how a bed bureau is perceived by referring GPs (and other doctors), is clarification of the role of a bed manager in finding a bed (with full authority to do that) and separating out the clinical component of the referral telephone call, which should be with clinical members of the 'on take' team, free of concern over practicalities of bed availability.

5.5.3.3 Bed availability Some concern was expressed over 'bed-blocking' by keeping beds occupied by patients, ready for discharge, until the next 'on take' day to ensure that beds would be available then for the new intake, and protection of elective beds, informally through similar 'bed-blocking' until the next surgical list, or formally by 'ring-fencing' some beds for GP fundholding practices or for other financially rewarding contracts (possibly extra-district contracts).

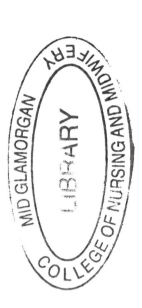

5.5.3.4 Admissions wards No hospital admitted all GP referrals direct to wards but for nearly two-thirds this was the principal route and no hospital admitted all GP referrals via central admissions units or accident and emergency departments but for nearly one-third this was the principal route. There were specialties (e.g. paediatrics and gynaecology) that usually took the 'direct' route and orthopaedics usually took the accident and emergency route. The main inter-hospital variation was with respect to admissions procedures for the principal admitting specialties of medicine, surgery and geriatrics and the accompanying medical or surgical specialities (e.g. cardiology or urology). Advantages were described for both systems, the preference often depended on geography and layout of hospital (or hospitals) and the size of specialties. Nearly half the hospitals visited had admissions wards, ranging from single specialty (medicine or surgery) wards with possibly very rapid turnover (stay ranging between 4 and 24 hours) to shared specialty wards taking many urgent referrals for their first 24-48 hours. While some criticisms of the admission ward concept were voiced, including postponing decision as to whether or not to admit, indecision as to which specialty to admit to and possible infrequency of visits by consultants, such criticisms were few.

Admissions wards were generally seen to have the major advantage of concentrating diagnostic and therapeutic activity on new arrivals in one place with higher nurse staffing levels and with appropriate equipment for treatment of seriously or critically ill patients. This allows housemen on admitting teams, particularly those in major specialties, to spend all (or most) of their 'on take' day in one area. It also has advantages for the principal diagnostic services if most of the urgent requests come from and return to a centralised admissions ward.

5.5.3.5 Observation wards Relatively few hospitals visited had observation wards, associated with accident and emergency departments. The role for such wards with relatively low nurse staffing for certain classes of patient was fairly clearly stated and several accident and emergency departments advised that development of observation wards ranked highly in their 'plans for change'. When hospital layout is appropriate, some day surgery units have been used for this purpose.

5.5.3.6 Seniority of admitting doctor The broad issue of who first sees urgent and emergency admissions was discussed at several visits. It is accepted that for many urgent patients, the need for admission has been assessed by the referring GP (or other doctor) and that therefore the principal role of the accepting doctor is 'clerking'. However, a significant number (though possibly a small number) of GP referrals are seriously or critically ill and require the early attention of senior and experienced doctors. Additionally, for a significant number of urgent admissions the need for admission is not well defined, the diagnosis uncertain and the ensuing clinical decision-making demands knowledge and experience of a more senior doctor. For these patients the appropriateness of using the most junior doctors (house officers of even medical students) to assess and diagnose has been questioned. Delays in initial treatment, first clinical action or admission can occur, while the house officer is observing or deliberating or awaiting more senior advice. This practice also leads to a certain number of 'inappropriate' admissions who are discharged at the next ward round by a more senior and experienced doctor but who might have been saved admission if they had been seen first by the more senior and experienced. Assessment of need for admission by a house officer of (emergency) patients referred through the accident and emergency department has been described as inappropriate, since the need for admission has already been assessed by a more senior doctor in the accident and emergency department.

5.5.3.7 Communication Weakness in inter-specialty communication was cited by several hospitals as contributing to difficulties in urgent admissions. Few hospitals described written protocols or agreed criteria for inter-specialty or inter-hospital transfer, but many thought that these could aid inter- specialty understanding and speed up inter-specialty transfer. The most frequently described difficulties for accident and emergency departments were for psychiatric admissions, often because the whole of the psychiatric service, including 'on call' team, was remote from the hospital at which the accident and emergency department was situated. Doctors who are not regularly working with mentally ill patients are unlikely to have the experience to manage these patients and may perceive a need to act conservatively because of the Mental Health Act (1983). Few of the hospitals visited had appropriate facilities for violent or disturbed patients in the accident and emergency department or readily accessible 'liaison psychiatrists' expediting arrangements for the rapid transfer of psychiatric patients away from accident and emergency departments. A Royal College of Physicians working party is currently reviewing this aspect of inter-specialty communication (Roy. Col. Phys. and Psych., 1993).

5.5.4 Liaison

5.5.4.1 Liaison with GPs All hospitals were conscious of the importance of communication between GPs and specialists, to achieve good quality referrals and hence to make the most appropriate use of acute hospital beds. It was also appreciated that good communication was two way and that to maintain good continuity of care at discharge (after acute admission) GPs need in their turn early advice of what the hospital is doing. Communication between GPs and hospital doctors varied widely between hospitals visited, from the "them and us" to good co-operation with many GPs regularly attending and taking leading roles in their local post-graduate education centres and in some districts being actively involved in hospital management.

5.5.4.2 Liaison with Social Services and community care The importance of discharge planning 'from the time of admission' was appreciated in most hospitals, although few reported having a discharge liaison co-ordinator. Audits have shown that many bed days are taken up by patients clinically ready for discharge but for whom some community care or social service has not been confirmed (Farag 1985). Some hospitals considered that 'Care in the community' has impeded discharge. Many hospitals kept a running tally of the number of beds blocked by patients they wished to discharge but could not, because appropriate arrangements had not been made in community care: in several large hospitals as many as 10% of acute beds were occupied by such patients. Most hospitals felt that better discharge planning and a higher profile for the 'discharge planner' could free many beds for new urgent (and elective) referrals.

5.5.5 Other Issues

5.5.5.1 Admission 'rights' Following discussion of the appropriateness of house officers in admitting teams examining patients to 'approve' admission after the need for admission had been ascertained by more senior and experienced staff (in accident and emergency departments) (see section 7.5.3.5), the issue of accident and emergency admission 'rights' was raised in several hospitals. In some, it appeared that the accident and emergency departments were allowed such rights informally, while in others accident and emergency staff remained frustrated that admissions could only be 'approved' by members of the 'on take' firm, however junior. This was perceived as a particular anomaly for a consultant-led specialty, when by comparison direct referrals by GPs were effectively admitted (at least for 24 hours or up until the next routine ward round) since house officers seldom took responsibility for 'discharging' a patient referred by a GP. A few accident and emergency departments had arrangements for temporary admission, for example for observation of head injuries or overnight for a patient fit for discharge on clinical grounds but kept in because of the hour and possible unsuitability of domestic or social arrangements. An area that was used in several hospitals for such temporary admissions was the day surgery unit, if convenient to the accident and emergency department.

5.5.5.2 'Hostel' beds A number of suggestions were made for change in use or allocation of beds, which may be regarded as extensions of practice already tried in some of the hospitals visited. One is the establishment of 'hostel' beds for convalescing patients prior to discharge. Recognition that some patients require less in the way of nursing care would allow redeployment of nursing allocation away from these wards to work with more acutely ill patients on admissions wards. It is possible also that 'hostel' beds could be used for certain short stay patients admitted more for social than clinical reasons and whose nursing requirements were minimal.

5.5.5.3 Bed 'ownership' Since in the final analysis 'beds are for patients and not for consultants', the more radical suggestion was for change of 'ownership' of beds. Several hospitals described use of pooled beds in admissions wards shared by several specialties and others described formalised arrangements for 'borrowing' beds that could be operated by the bed manager, which effectively pools beds when demand exceeded supply in one of the admitting specialties. It is a relatively short step practically from there to developing a more general formula for the use of beds throughout the acute specialties. (Audit Commission 1992).

5.5.5.4 Information technology/Communication aids Few hospitals were making full use of modern electronic communication systems, including portable telephones and fax (and possibly electronic mail), for example for ECG, X-ray and laboratory reports. More widespread use of such systems could bring both consultant and the specialist diagnostic services closer to the patient and could speed up important clinical decisions. One practical suggestion that could help communication in many hospitals was for the introduction of mobile phones for consultants and fax machines in their offices. These are now relatively cheap and their use could provide junior doctors with more rapid advice, which in turn could lead to earlier treatment or admission for urgent and emergency patients.

5.5.5.5 Contracts for urgent and emergency admissions Almost all hospitals visited raised the issue of the funding formula and the balance between urgent and elective patients. The hospital view (clinicians, clinical directors and managers) was almost invariably that rewards were for treating elective patients and that the desirable contracts to negotiate with purchasing authorities were those for the more adventurous 'regional' specialties. While hospitals are under an obligation to treat urgent and emergency patients and while provision is made in the funding formula for treating these, the widespread feeling of the providers was that, by fulfilling their statutory and moral obligations to patients, they were not being adequately or appropriately rewarded. A more satisfactory balance in the funding formula should be struck so that hospitals are rewarded rather than penalised for treating urgent and emergency patients.

5.5.5.6 Urgent and emergency hospital care in 21st century

All hospitals were mindful of possible gains in efficiency that could be made and how new medical techniques can lead to better use of resources. Nevertheless many hospitals wished to register a concern over the need to maintain adequate health care resources in urgent and emergency services, particularly in medical and nursing staff who work directly with patients, to minimise any possible risk of unsafe understaffing (UK Health Ministers 1986), to meet standards that are currently being set in contract negotiations and to improve standards in the future "to raise the performance of all hospitals and GP practices to that of the best" (Secretary of State for Health 1989). It was felt important to consider resource needs within the context of increasing numbers of admissions to hospital (Office of Population Censuses and Surveys 1993) and of the increasing needs of an ageing society (Office of Population Censuses and Surveys 1991) which "the Government recognises will lead to a greater demand for services" (Secretary of State for Health 1991).

Chapter 6

Summary

6.1   Key admission times

Key times 'from arrival to doctor attending', 'from arrival to first clinical action', 'from arrival to admission' and 'from arrival to definitive management' varied widely. Admission times were slower in almost all hospitals in the South East (the four Thames health regions and the three regions bordering Greater London) than elsewhere in the UK. Reasons for this include differences in specialty requirements and physical layout of hospitals, but these are not sufficient to explain the extent of variation.

6.2   'Target' admission times

In more than half of the study hospitals, 80% or more of all urgent or emergency patients were seen by a doctor within 1 hour. Furthermore more than half of the study hospitals admitted 90% or more of their patients within four hours of arrival in hospital. These could be regarded as guidelines for setting standards. It should be possible to ensure that few patients wait more than an hour after arrival to be seen, or more than four hours for admission.

6.3   28 day outcome

An association was found between admission times and 28 day outcome: hospitals that were slow to admit tended to record higher 28 day death rates. Possible explanations for this association, which may include an (unwritten) policy of admitting terminal patients leading to high (population based) admission rates in turn leading to congestion and delay in admission, are being further investigated by the research team.

6.4   Best practice

Hospital visits (and questionnaires) revealed widely differing policies for management of urgent and emergency admission, and enabled better practices to be identified. While different situations may require different solutions in detail, many features of urgent and emergency admissions are common to all hospitals and many 'best practices' are relevant to most situations. These are summarised briefly as follows.

6.5 Admission management

Hospitals frequently described problems in finding beds for urgent or emergency admissions. This sometimes reflects a shortage of beds, but more often it is because beds are unstaffed or unavailable (for a particular patient in the appropriate specialty at that time).

6.6 Bed ownership

Some hospitals have taken practical steps to improve bed management and patient turn-over, by moving away from the tradition of 'consultant ownership' of beds and towards pooling beds and managing beds in groups. The Audit Commission has recommended this development (Audit Commission 1992).

6.7 Admission wards

Admission wards are in use in several hospitals. These enable high dependency nursing establishment to be available for all acutely ill patients. The forms these wards take varies from hospital to hospital; they may be single specialty or multi-specialty and either single or mixed gender. They provide flexibility and minimise disturbance to other patients. It is important to plan sufficient capacity to accommodate peak demands to avoid disrupting elective services. This may be achieved by having extra beds available and staffing them when necessary.

6.8 Observation wards in accident and emergency departments

A few hospitals have observation wards associated with accident and emergency departments. These are used with low dependency nursing establishment for short stay patients, such as those retained for social reasons. Some conveniently situated day surgery units, which are otherwise vacant at night, are used for this purpose. Further analysis of data obtained in this study is directed towards assessing the potential for observation wards.

6.9 Emergency operating theatres

It has been recommended previously that emergency theatres should be available 24 hours a day (Buck 1987). Despite this recommendation emergency theatres are still not available 24 hours a day in many hospitals; or, if theatres are available, staff (anaesthetists, surgeons, nurses, technicians and ancillary) may not be. This contributes to delay and affects quality of emergency services.

6.10 Bed closures

Closing beds, when elective admissions are curtailed or for financial reasons, reduces flexibility for emergencies. Both urgent and elective admissions may be affected and protective measures may be employed by clinicians to retain patients in hospital to ensure admission of urgent patients in need or elective patients when planned. Such problems can be mitigated when there is close consultation with continuing dialogue between managers and clinicians.

6.11 Bed managers

Several hospitals have found bed managers successful in preventing 'log jams' and in reducing delays. They are only effective if they are given the necessary authority and seniority, work to agreed protocols and have the support of senior medical 'referees' or access to senior management. It is also important that they are available on a 24 hour basis.

6.12 'Hostel' or 'hotel' beds

It has been suggested that 'hostel' or 'hotel' beds could be useful for some patients, who are sufficiently recovered to be almost self-caring and who require minimal nursing care but who cannot be discharged for other reasons (e.g. social). The use of beds in this way could release other inpatient beds for more acutely ill patients and allow better deployment of nursing time. 'Hostel' beds, or minimal dependency nursing beds, may be obtained by partially reopening a closed ward even if only at times of peak demand.

6.13 Clinical directorates - communication and management

Clinical directorates (where established) seem to be effective in achieving better collaboration between specialties and in integrating use of resources for the emergency services. This emphasises the importance of involving clinicians in resource management.

6.14 Information technology - communications within hospital

Difficulty in contacting medical staff explained some delays in managing patients.

A few hospitals have improved communications with consultants on call by use of personal portable telephones and fax machines for, for example, ECG, X-ray and laboratory results. Information technology including personal telephones, fax and possibly electronic mail could be used more widely.

6.15 Availability of support services

In some hospitals relevant support and diagnostic services were not available and some relevant services were not called upon, because of budgetary constraints. Furthermore delays in obtaining diagnostic and other support services were the explanations for some delayed admissions. While some shortfall and some delays may be well known to clinicians and managers, others may not become apparent until times of obtaining these services are audited.

6.16 Discharge planning

Discharge planning should start at the time of admission with early social service involvement (when necessary). A discharge co-ordinator has been found helpful in some hospitals to facilitate this process particularly with difficult cases and particularly where communication between health and social services is difficult (see 5.6.24).

6.17 Hospital layout and design

'Split-site', 'multi-site' and even 'single-site' hospitals with widely dispersed wards create difficulty for staffing, requiring simultaneously available parallel teams. Several hospitals have inherited and adapted layouts that are inappropriate to modern acute medical practice. The possibility of concentrating all acute specialties on a single site should be considered; possible gains in effectiveness and efficiency of a single hospital, specifically designed for modern medical practice, might allow recovery of capital costs over a relatively short period.

6.18 Medical Staffing

Some accident and emergency departments do not yet have a consultant trained in accident and emergency medicine. Furthermore medical staffing levels in some accident and emergency departments were below recommendations and inadequate for the work-load, which may affect quality of care and lead to delays for emergency admissions. There are difficulties in increasing levels because of shortages of trained staff and restrictions on training.

6.19 Arrangements for admission via accident and emergency departments

A patient who has been referred by a consultant-led accident and emergency department and who clearly requires admission (e.g. fractured femur) should not have to wait for a further examination by a junior trainee before proceeding with admission. This practice, quite widespread, is wasteful of resources and causes delays to admission and treatment and distress to patients.

6.20 General practitioners

Some general practices have difficulty in providing a 24 hour service. This can lead to greater activity in accident and emergency departments and in turn delays in admission, not only for urgent patients arising from these practices but also for other patients.

6.21 Demand for 'primary care'

Some hospitals reported many patients seeking "primary care" in accident and emergency departments. Various methods have been and are being evaluated to alleviate such pressures in accident and emergency departments. One way is for general practitioners to manage such "primary care" patients, which allows accident and emergency staff to spend more time treating accident and emergency patients.

6.22 Nurse and other professional staffing

Shortages explained delays in establishing formal triage in many accident and emergency departments, some emergency theatre non-availability, and (out of hours) delays in obtaining diagnostic services. It has been noted previously that nurse staffing levels in general owe more to history than to evaluation of patient need (Audit Commission 1991).

6.23 Nurse practitioners

Nurse practitioners are employed in few accident and emergency departments. Their role could usefully be explored and evaluated more fully.

6.24 Psychiatric patients in accident and emergency

'Care in the Community' (Secretary of State for Health 1981) has led to an increase in use of accident and emergency departments by patients with psychiatric problems. Appropriate care and admission of these patients is often aggravated by siting all psychiatric services away from the accident and emergency department (and district general hospital). Care for these patients, some of whom may require a great deal of attention, also diverts resources from attending to other urgent patients. Liaison between accident and emergency departments and psychiatry could ease these burdens. There should be a psychiatric presence in the district general hospital.

6.25 Discharge and social services

Bed availability for urgent and emergency admissions depends on ability to discharge. Most hospitals have beds occupied by patients awaiting social services or community care. There appear to be few time standards for assessment and fewer for implementation of the care package. Delays in approving and obtaining appropriate social services or community care can give rise to significant delays in discharge. A study is currently under way to investigate these issues and address these problems (Department of Health 1993).

6.26 Resource implications

Addressing many of these issues, as in the following recommendations, may well be resource neutral and achieved by rearrangement of existing resources and improvements in efficiency. Nevertheless "raising the performance of all hospitals — to that of the best" (Secretary of State for Health 1991) with respect to urgent and emergency admissions, which account for over half of all hospital admissions, may have resource implications in some districts.

6.27 NHS reforms and services for urgent and emergency admissions

There was no direct evidence in the timing study to suggest that the NHS reforms had affected services for urgent and emergency admissions (either way) but there are no comparable timing data from pre-reform days and the impact of some of these reforms are only beginning to emerge. To assess whether or not the NHS reforms affect timeliness of urgent or emergency services another study will be needed in about two years time.

6.28 'Community care' and services for urgent and emergency admissions

The Community Care Act has been introduced rapidly and it will take time for new working practices to become established. This study finds that the Community Care Act has affected urgent and emergency admissions and discharges, which affect bed availability (as outlined above). These effects may be short term: to establish the longer term effects of the Community Care Act on urgent and emergency admissions a further study will be required after new intersectoral relationships have become established.

6.29 Review of services for urgent and emergency admission

Many changes in management and practice of health and social services and community care have been introduced in a very short period of time. Some of these changes will almost certainly affect emergency services, but the effects of these Acts, changes and reforms are only beginning to be felt. To monitor effects of the emergency services, it will be necessary to undertake both audit locally and further review nationally.

Chapter 7

Recommendations

Our recommendations are based on (i) Analysis of information obtained in the study of urgent or emergency admission in 30 representative hospitals across the country (ii) Reports of the doctors supervising the data gathering study in each hospital (iii) Answers to the questionnaires completed by study hospitals (iv) Visits to all hospitals by committee members (v) Discussion with senior managers and clinicians at all hospitals and (vi) Deliberation within the full committee and with professional colleagues. We recommend that:

7.1   Standards

7.1.1   **National guidelines should be developed for the emergency services under the auspices of the Royal Colleges and the Health Departments.** These should relate to timeliness (e.g. >80% seen by a doctor within one hour or >90% admitted within four hours) and inter-alia to access, availability, effectiveness and quality. **These should be incorporated into standards agreed in local protocols and contracts by purchasing authorities.**

7.1.2   A library of policy documents on emergency services, which have been developed or are being developed in regions and districts, by specialist associations and by Royal Colleges, should be collated by the Health Departments and be accessible to NHS regions, districts and trusts.

7.2   Contracting for urgent and emergency services

7.2.1   **Purchasers should contract for and hospitals should receive appropriate funding for the provision of emergency services according to activity and quality in order to balance the present contracting system which tends to encourage elective services.**

7.2.2   **Contracts should provide, to a greater extent than at present, for variations in demand which may arise in time (seasonally or daily in the travelling population) and in place (characteristics of the population and cross boundary flow).**

7.2.3   **Hospitals' management must give the necessary priority to emergency services.**

7.2.4 **Initiatives such as those to reduce elective waiting lists should be implemented in a way that does not adversely affect the emergency services.**

7.2.5 **Necessary resource implications should be addressed.** Many of the recommendations in this report will be 'resource neutral', and achievable by rearrangements of existing resources and improvements in efficiency, but some may have resource implications in some districts.

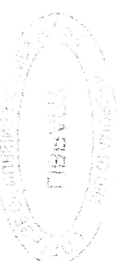

7.3   Admission times

Health authorities (purchasers) should examine their arrangements and hospitals (providers) should examine their procedures urgently to seek necessary improvements in timing of key events in the admission of urgent or emergency patients.

7.4   Admission management

Hospitals should review the management arrangements for urgent or emergency admission including consideration of the following:-

7.4.1   Bed ownership

The move away from traditional 'consultant ownership' of beds and towards development of schemes of bed pooling for the appropriate care of urgent and emergency admissions.

7.4.2   Admission wards

The use of admission wards in some form and further operational research into their optimum organisation.

7.4.3   Observation wards in accident and emergency departments

To the introduction of observation wards in some form and further operational research to identify the best modes of organising them.

7.4.4   Emergency operating theatres

Urgent moves to provide 24 hour availability of emergency theatres.

7.4.5   Bed closures

Collaboration of managers and clinicians to address problems in the emergency services which result from reduced bed capacity when bed closures are necessary.

7.4.6 Bed managers

The appointment of bed managers with appropriate authority and seniority to operate a 24 hour service within agreed protocols.

7.4.7 'Hostel' or 'hotel' beds

Operational research to evaluate the role of 'hostel' or 'hotel' beds and to develop these ideas in the most efficient manner.

7.4.8 Clinical directorates - communication and management

The further development of clinical directorates to ensure the full and continuing collaboration of managers and clinicians in use of resources for emergency services.

7.4.9 Information technology - communications within hospital

Exploration of potential uses of information technology to facilitate the rapid transfer of relevant information (results of diagnostic tests) and improve communication with consultants on call.

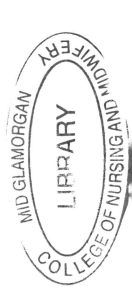

7.4.10 Staffing

Review of nursing and other professional staffing and distribution to meet needs of emergency services.

7.4.11 Availability of support services

Audit of availability and times of obtaining diagnostic and other supporting services to identify shortfalls and delays.

7.4.12 Discharge planning

The appointment of discharge co-ordinators.

7.5 Organisation of services for urgent and emergency admission

7.5.1 Hospital layout and design:

When acute care is provided on split- or multiple-sites, consideration should be given to placing all acute specialties on a single site.

7.5.2 Consultant-led accident and emergency departments:

7.5.2.1 **All accident and emergency departments should be led by a consultant, trained in accident and emergency medicine.**

7.5.2.2 **Inadequate medical establishment should be resolved by the Health Departments and the Royal Colleges by increasing number of training posts.**

7.5.2.3 **Hand-over arrangements should be agreed so that patients may be admitted without repeated examination by junior trainees (from other departments).**

7.5.3 General Practitioners

7.5.3.1 **Problems that some general practices have in providing a 24 hour service should be addressed by F.H.S.A.s.**

7.5.3.2 Further studies should be undertaken to address the issue of demand for 'primary care' in some accident and emergency departments.

7.5.4 Nurse practitioners

Further evaluation of nurse practitioner schemes in accident and emergency should be undertaken.

7.5.5 Psychiatric patients in accident and emergency

Substantive arrangements should be developed in consultation with psychiatrists to deal with problems associated with psychiatric patients in accident and emergency departments.

7.5.6 Discharge and social services

Solutions should be sought urgently to counter discharge delays attributable to Social Services or Community Care.

7.5.7 'Community care' and services for urgent and emergency admissions

Closer consultation should be developed between separate sectors of health, social and community care to ensure the desirable 'seamless' service.

7.6 Review of services for accident and emergency admission

7.6.1 Hospital audit

Hospitals should conduct regular audits of issues raised in this Report.

7.6.2 National review

A further national review of urgent and emergency admission should be undertaken in two years' time.

References

1.   Secretary of State for Health, Wales, Northern Ireland and Scotland. Working for patients. HMSO. London 1989.

2.   Department of Health. The Patient's Charter. HMSO. London 1991.

3.   Royal College of Surgeons. Report of working party on management of patients with the major injuries. RCS London 1988.

4.   British Association for Accident and Emergency Medicine. Medical staffing in accident and emergency departments. BAEM. London 1991.

5.   Department of Health. Welfare of children and young people in hospital. HMSO. London 1991.

6.   National Audit Office. NHS accident and emergency departments in England. HMSO London 1992.

7.   Scottish Health Management Efficiency Group. Multi-disciplinary group on accident and emergency services. Edinburgh 1992.

8.   Yorkshire Health Authority. Principles for emergency and urgent care in Yorkshire. YHA, Harrogate 1992.

9.   Dale J., Green J., Glucksman E R., Higgs R. Providing for primary care, progress in accident and emergency departments. Kings College Hospital, London. 1991.

10.   Department of Health. Charter standards in the NHS. HMSO. London 1992.

11.   Office of Population Census and Surveys. Hospital inpatient enquiry (1979-85). HMSO. London 1981-88.

12.   Milner P.C., Nichol J.P., Williams B.T. Variation in demand for accident and emergency departments in England from 1974 to 1985. J. Epid. Comm. Health. 1991. 42. 274-78.

13.   Office of Population Census and Surveys. Hospital episode statistics (for year 1989- 90). HMSO. London 1993.

14.   Champion H.R., Sacco W.J., Copes W.S., Gann D.S., Gennarelli T.A., Flanagan M.E. A revision of the trauma score. J Trauma 1989; 29. 623-9.

15.   Mathey D.G., Sheehan F., Schofer J., Dodge H.T. Time from onset of symptoms to thrombolytic therapy; a major determinant of myocardial salvage in patients with acute transmural infarction. J Am Coll Cardiol 1985. 6. 518-25.

16.   ISIS-2 (Second International Study of Infarct Survival). Collaborative Group. A multicentre, randomised trial of intravenous streptokinase and aspirin in acute myocardial infarction. Lancet 1988; ii. 349-60.

17. CMA Medical data. Directory of emergency and special care units. CM Medical Data, Cambridge. 1992.

18. Royal College of General Practitioners. Morbidity statistics from general practice second national study 1970-71. Studies on medical and population subjects - 26. HMSO. London 1974.

19. Jones D.A., Cranton S. Study of discharge from hospital and aftercare of older persons who were urgent admissions. Clinical Standards Advisory Group, Dept of Health, London, 1993.

20. Jones D.A., Lester C., West R.R. Monitoring changes in health services for older people. (Chapter). Kings Fund. London 1993.

21. Roy. Colls. Phys. and Psych. Joint working party on psychiatry liaison. (Chair Dawson A.) Roy. Colls. Phys. and Psych. London 1993.

22. Farag R.R., Tinker G.M., Delay in discharge of patients from an acute geriatric unit. Health Trends. 1985. 17. 41.

23. Audit Commission. Lying in wait: the use of medical beds in acute hospitals. HMSO, London 1992.

24. Office of Population Censuses and Surveys. National population projections 1989 based. Series, PP 2, no. 17. HMSO, London 1991.

25. British Association for Accident and Emergency Medicine. The way ahead: accident and emergency services 2001. BAEM, London 1992.

26. Secretary of State for Health. NHS and community care act. HMSO, London 1990.

27. Department of Health. Care in the community: consultation document on moving resources for care in England. Department of Health. HMSO, London 1981.

28. Secretary of State for Health. Mental Health Act, 1983. HMSO, London 1983.

29. Secretary of State for Health. Health of the Nation. HMSO, London 1991.

30. UK Health Department, joint consultative committee, chairman of regional health authorities. Hospital medical staffing; achieving a balance. D.H.S.S. London 1986.

31. Department of Health. Health building note 22, Accident and Emergency Departments. HMSO, London 1988.

32. Buck N., Devlin B.V., Lunn J.N. Report of confidential inquiry into perioperative deaths. Nuffield. Prov. Hosp. Trust. London 1987.

33. Audit Commission. Virtue of patients: making best use of ward nursing resources. HMSO. London. 1991.

34. Department of Health Social Services Inspectorate. Special project on "December 31st agreements". DoH. London 1993.

Glossary

Glossary for purposes of CSAG study of urgent or emergency admission to hospital)

Single-site hospital: most of 'district' acute specialties including accident and emergency department available on one site. (Note: a 'single-site hospital' (or trust) may not be the only hospital providing normal DGH specialties in a district).

Split-site hospital: (usually) two hospitals or a two-site hospital providing together most of 'district' acute specialties with transfers from the accident and emergency department (on one site) to specialties (on another) or between specialties (on different sites) commonplace.

'District' acute specialties: include all main specialties expected of a DGH but exclude 'regional' specialties (like cardiac surgery, burns and plastic surgery) for which transfers would be expected from most DGHs.

Emergency: 999 ambulance, immediate.

Urgent GP referral: seeks admission immediately or within hours (note: includes requests from deputising services).

Self referral: includes walk in, urgent self-referral on prior arrangement or understanding (e.g. asthma or cardiac patient) and emergency when ambulance not used (e.g. for children).

Other (urgent) referral: principally inter-specialty referrals, inter-hospital referrals, referrals from out patients, day hospital or domiciliary visits.

Admissions Unit: a reception area dedicated to clinical clerking of urgent admissions by receiving teams or 'on take' firms, in the style of an accident and emergency department with patients on trolleys in bays (Assessment Unit).

Admission Ward: a short stay (24 hour) ward for the reception, early treatment and observation of urgent admissions by receiving teams, usually with relatively few beds (8-12), high nurse staffing and cleared daily by ward round of appropriate receiving teams (or 'on take' firms). (24 hour ward/observation ward).

Direct admissions: attended first by medical staff of specialist receiving team or 'on take' firm, whether on ward, in admissions ward or in admissions unit (which may be staffed by nurses from accident and emergency).

Indirect admissions: attended first by accident and emergency medical staff and therefore requiring 'referral' to appropriate specialty and 'reclerking' by receiving team or 'on take' firm (compare 'direct' admissions).

Other terms are used in conventional sense and are not crucial to understanding the findings of this report.

Study hospitals

APPENDIX 2. Study Hospitals

1.   Darlington Memorial Hospital, 552 beds
        Darlington DHA, Northern RHA
        Pop. 124,500

2.   Gateshead, Queen Elizabeth Hospital, 503 beds
        Gateshead DHA, Northern RHA
        Pop. 206,900

3.   Halifax General/Halifax Royal Infirmary, 427/244 beds
        Calderdale DHA, Yorkshire RHA
        Pop. 195,900

4.   Bradford Royal Infirmary/St Luke's Hospital, 664/463 beds
        (Bradford Hospitals NHS Trust)
        Bradford DHA, Yorkshire RHA
        Pop. 340,000

5.   Chesterfield & North Derbyshire Royal Hospital, 718 beds
        North Derbyshire HA, Trent RHA
        Pop. 363,200

6.   i)   Royal Hallamshire Hospital, 728 beds
             (Central Sheffield University Hospital NHS Trust)
        ii) Sheffield Childrens Hospital NHS Trust, 159 beds
        iii) Sheffield Northern General Hospital NHS Trust, 1041 beds
             Sheffield DHA, Trent RHA
             Pop. 526,000

7.   Addenbrooke's Hospital, Cambridge, 845 beds
        Cambridge HA, East Anglia RHA
        Pop. 282,880

8.   Northwick Park Hospital, Harrow, 600 beds
        Harrow HA, NW Thames RHA
        Pop. 192,500

9.   Lister Hospital, Stevenage, 391 beds
        North Herts NHS Trust
        North Herts HA, NW Thames RHA
        Pop. 186,000

10. University College Hospital, London, 398 beds
    Bloomsbury & Islington HA, NE Thames RHA
    Pop. 291,123

11. Broomfield Hospital, Chelmsford, 332 beds
    (Mid Essex Hospitals NHS Trust)
    Mid Essex HA, NE Thames RHA
    Pop. 290,800

12. King's College Hospital, 557 beds
    (King's Healthcare Trust)
    Camberwell HA, SE Thames RHA
    Pop. 210,500

13. Eastbourne District General Hospital, 742 beds
    (Eastbourne Hospitals NHS Trust)
    Eastbourne DHA, SE Thames
    Pop. 235,200

14. Kingston Hospital Trust, 520 beds
    Kingston & Esher HA, SW Thames
    Pop. 180,800

15. Southampton General Hospital/Royal South Hampshire Hospital,
    888/348 beds
    Southampton & SW Hants DHA, Wessex RHA
    Pop. 419,700

16. Royal Berkshire Hospital/Battle Hospital, Reading, 551/398 beds
    West Berkshire HA, Oxford RHA,
    Pop. 466,700

17. Taunton & Somerset Hospital (Trust), 604 beds
    One of two acute hospitals in Somerset HA, South Western RHA
    Pop. 412,500

18. Southmead Hospital, Bristol, 650 beds
    (Southmead Health Services NHS Trust)
    Southmead HA, South Western RHA
    Pop. 232,300

19. City General Hospital/North Staffordshire Royal Infirmary, 569/509 beds
    North Staffs HA, West Midlands RHA
    Pop. 461,000

20. The Royal Hospital/New Cross Hospital, Wolverhampton, 195/510 beds
    Wolverhampton HA, West Midlands RHA
    Pop. 250,000

21. Southport & Formby District General Hospital (Trust), 307 beds
    Southport & Formby DHA, Mersey RHA
    Pop. 120,773

22. Bolton General Hospital/Bolton Royal Infirmary, 826/233 beds
    Bolton HA, North Western RHA
    Pop. 263,700

23. i) Withington Hospital, 1117 beds
    ii) Wythenshawe Hospital, Manchester, 901 beds
        South Manchester HA, North Western RHA
        Pop. 183,800

24. i) Royal Gwent Hospital 617 beds
    ii) Nevil Hall Hospital, 421 beds
        Gwent HA, Wales
        Pop. 446,800

25. The Ayr Hospital, 301 beds
    South Ayrshire Hospitals NHS Trust
    One of three acute hospitals in Ayrshire & Arran HB, Scotland
    Pop. 374,443

26. Ninewells Hospital/Royal Infirmary, Dundee, 793/288 beds
    Tayside HB, Scotland
    Pop. 393,762

27. Coleraine Hospital, NI, 211 beds
    One of three acute hospitals in Northern HB, Northern Ireland
    Pop. 374,600

Timing record sheet

UK STUDY OF URGENT OR EMERGENCY ADMISSION TO HOSPITAL

PATIENT LABEL

Name:
Address:

Hospital No:
Date of birth:

district/hospital

study number (patient)

999=1, bed bureau=2, other ....

date

TIME

Patient (or proxy) request

GP request

Ambulance on scene <

Reason for delay (if significant)[1] ....

Accident and Emergency/Receiving station/Ward arrival

Primary management

Medical officer attends

Doctor[3] .... grade ....

Reason for delay (if sig)[1] ....

Provisional diagnosis[4] ....

Investigation[5] ....

Treatment[6] ....

Initial treatment (decision to refer to admitting team)

(Seen by admitting team)

Reason for delay (if sig)[1] ....

Admission to definitive ward/specialty[7]

Definitive management

Specialty[8] ....

Reason for delay (if sig)[1] ....

Definitive management begins

Doctor[9] .... grade ....

Reason for delay (if sig)[1] ....

Investigation[5] ....

Treatment[10] ....

....

PLEASE RETURN TO EMERGENCY ADMISSIONS (Attn of: ....)
and finally to Dr R R West, University of Wales College of Medicine,
Heath Park, Cardiff, CF4 4XN.

final diagnosis[11] ....

principal clinical actions ....

additional to above[12] ....

total stay (days)

disposal (hospital, hosp other spec, other hosp, home, conv hosp, dead)[13]

28 day outcome

Times (24 hour clock). If next day write new date alongside.

1. Significant delay: guide 1 hour but if truly urgent shorter delays
    may be significant.

2. Time of arrival in hospital, whether A&E, receiving station or
    direct to (definitive) ward. The form allows for one 'temporary'
    (primary) location before admission to 'definitive' treatment: if
    more than one 'temporary' location start second form here and
    staple to first form.

3. Medical Officer, the doctor who first attends patient after
    arrival (not literally "first to see", e.g. if serious and a
    senior arrives promptly and takes responsibility. Enter name
    (caps please) and grade, (HO, SHO, Reg, Sen Reg, Clin Asst, Locum
    Cons, Cons).

4. Provisional diagnosis. Enter clearly (eg severe chest pain? AMI).

5. Investigation. Enter (eg X-ray).

6. Treatment, emergency or primary (in A&E, receiving ward). Enter
    (eg. streptokinase)

7. Admission: planned stay at least until next ward round. The form
    allows for one definitive specialty: if more than one start second
    form here for second specialty and staple to first form.

8. Enter specialty (ward and hospital, as appropriate).

9. The doctor who starts definitive management, (see 3 above).

10. Definitive management. Enter important treatments (eg.
    defibrillation, CPR, lignocaine): if further urgent or emergency
    definitive treatment in another specialty (ward) start new form at
    7 (see 7 above), if further non-urgent treatment in another
    secialty/hospital see 28 day outcome (12 below).

11. Principal diagnosis, that led to this admission. Supervisor will

12. Further clinical actions, relevant to urgent or emergency
    conditions.

13. Disposal: at 28 days: hospital same specialty (whether or not
    discharged and readmitted) 1, hospital another specialty 2,
    transfer to another hospital 3, discharge home 4, convalescent
    home 5, died 6.

Age and sex of urgent and emergency admissions

Age group		Emergency (999)	Urgent GP	Self referral	Other	Not known	All admission
0-4	M	42	225	157	5	13	442
	F	41	190	117	6	8	362
5-	M	44	127	112	8	11	302
	F	33	94	63	4	2	196
15-	M	111	85	111	7	13	327
	F	91	188	107	5	9	400
25-	M	117	104	112	12	3	348
	F	73	198	91	17	13	392
35-	M	77	125	70	8	9	289
	F	64	113	75	10	7	269
45-	M	93	117	65	16	6	297
	F	65	116	37	7	5	306
55-	M	125	217	70	20	7	439
	F	73	175	43	10	5	306
65-	M	178	327	48	20	10	583
	F	147	284	43	14	5	493
75+	M	209	418	58	13	11	709
	F	342	633	82	18	12	1087
Not known	M	37	44	21	2	-	108
	F	35	67	14	2	-	122

Information on age or sex of patients was missing on 56 forms (1%) and information on admission route was missing on 213 forms (3%).

The number of males and females were similar. The elderly were rather more likely to be admitted as emergencies (999). Children were more likely to 'self refer' 'Other' urgent admissions included admissions from out patients, day hospital or domiciliaries, inter-specialty and inter-hospital transfers.

Grade of doctor
who first attends

	Emergency (999)	Urgent GP	Self referral	Other	All referrals
House Officer	154	1276	154	26	1632
SHO	1517	1993	1136	79	4828
Registrar	112	252	59	31	461
Sen Reg	12	19	7	1	39
Consultant	55	28	52	29	168
Other (staff grade)	33	24	18	2	77

Information on the grade of doctor or admission route was missing on 568 (7%) of patient forms.

Nearly two thirds of urgent and emergency referrals were seen first by an SHO; more than three quarters among emergency (999) and self referrals and about half among urgent GP referrals. Nearly one quarter were seen first by house officers, most commonly among urgent GP referrals. Those 999 emergency referrals and self-referrals seen first by house officers were mostly in admissions units or on wards (rather than in accident and emergency departments). About 7% were seen first by (senior) registrars, more commonly among the relatively few 'other' referrals, which were predominantly inter-hospital transfers or transfers from outpatient clinics. Only 2% were first seen by consultants, again more commonly among 'other' referrals.

Emergency Services Committee

Members

Professor Michael Rosen CBE, Department of Anaesthetics, University Hospital of Wales, CARDIFF - Chairman
(Past president Royal College of Anaesthetists), (Clinical Standards Advisory Group)*

Dr Stuart Carne CBE, FRCGP, 5 St Mary Abbots Court, Warwick Gardens, LONDON
(Past president Royal College of General Practitioners), (Clinical Standards Advisory Group)*

Dr Stephen Farrow MD,FFPHM, Director of Public Health, Barnet Health Agency, LONDON*

Miss Pam Hibbs OBE, FRCN, Chief Nurse, City & Hackney Health Authority, LONDON
(Chairman Standing Nursing & Midwifery Advisory Committee and Member of Clinical Standards Advisory Group to April 1993)*

Mr G Jones, Royal College of Nursing, LONDON

Dr John Lunn MD, FRCA, Department of Anaesthetics, University of Wales College of Medicine, CARDIFF
(Confidential enquiry into perioperative deaths)*

Mr Stephen Miles FRCS, Consultant in Accident and Emergency, St Bartholomew's and Homerton Hospitals, LONDON
(British Association for Accident and Emergency Medicine)*

Dr I J Nuala Sterling CBE, FRCP, Consultant Physician in Geriatric Medicine, Royal South Hants Hospital, SOUTHAMPTON
(Chairman Standing Medical Advisory Committee), (Clinical Standards Advisory Group)*

Research Director

Dr Robert West FSS, MFPHM hon, Reader in Epidemiology, University of Wales College of Medicine, CARDIFF*

Additional Members ("Sounding Board")

Professor Stuart Cobbe MD, FRCP, Department of Medical Cardiology, University of Glasgow, GLASGOW*

Mr Hamish Macdonald PhD, FRCOG, Medical Director/Consultant Obstetrician and Gynaecologist, St James' University Hospital, LEEDS

Professor Brian Rowlands MD, FRCS, FACS, Department of Surgery, Queen's University of Belfast, BELFAST*

Mr S Westaby BSC, MS, FRCS, Consultant in Cardiothracic Surgery, John Radcliffe Hospital, OXFORD

* Hospital Visitors

Research Team

University of Wales College of Medicine, Cardiff

Dr Robert West	Reader in Epidemiology
Mrs Sandra Cranton	Research Officer (July - October 1992)
Mr Vaughan Evans	Research Officer (November 1992 - October 1993)
Mr Michael Imana	Research Registrar (NW Thames)
Mr Conor Kelly	Research Registrar (Trent)
Mr Ian Kendall	Research Senior Registrar (Trent)
Mr Nigel Kidner	Research Registrar (Trent)
Mr Michael McCabe	Research Senior Registrar (Wales)

Acknowledgements

We gratefully acknowledge assistance of teams of research nurses, particularly team leaders in all hospitals, without whom the study would not have been possible in the time available, and managers, clinical directors, nurse managers, medical records officers, ambulance officers and particularly clinical directors of accident and emergency departments, who facilitate

Government Response to CSAG's Report on Urgent and Emergency Admissions to Hospitals

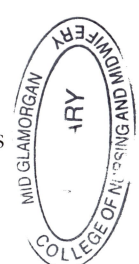

The Government welcomes the publication of CSAG's report on urgent and emergency admissions which will contribute to thinking in an important area of health provision. Copies of the report will be distributed to the relevant interests in the NHS.

Appropriate admission and discharge procedures being in place is a major quality of service issue and one which demands the attention of local managers. Health authorities are responsible for ensuring that hospitals with whom they contract have flexible systems in place that enable them to respond promptly to short term fluctuations in the emergency workload. The objective must be that patients are given a bed on a suitable ward as soon as possible after initial assessment and a decision to admit and that their dignity and comfort is maintained during any waiting period.

Many of CSAG's recommendations are directed at hospitals and health authorities and deal with details of service provision which are the responsibility of local management within the general policy framework outlined above. In these cases we have not thought it appropriate in the response to individual recommendations below to comment on the detail.

Standards

CSAG Recommendation:

7.1.1 National guidelines should be developed for the emergency services under the auspices of the Royal Colleges and the Health Department. These should relate to timeliness (eg >80% seen by a doctor within one hour or >90% admitted within four hours) and inter-alia to access, availability, effectiveness and quality. These should be incorporated into standards agreed in local protocols and contracts by purchasing authorities.

Government Response (to para 7.1.1):

We recognise that the need for the NHS to respond satisfactorily to the needs of patients presenting as emergencies, by whatever route, raises issues in many cases different from those raised in relation to pre-planned (ie elective) treatment and that the issues raised are the right ones. A number of relevant issues are raised in this report, and in other contexts, which we shall be considering. Among these latter, concerns have been expressed by the medical profession and others over an apparent rise in the number of emergency admissions as a proportion of all admissions. In response, the NHS Executive commissioned a study to examine changes in emergency admissions in 10 major hospitals. The study found that most of the apparent rise was due to movement of work from elective admissions to day cases, and that non-elective work as a proportion of all admissions (including day-cases) had remained steady, although there were local variations. No evidence was found of wide-scale changes in GP referral patterns (for either fundholders or non-fundholders). However we plan to look more closely at this issue. We have set up 4 demonstration sites to examine the balance of emergency to elective work and to look at ways of improving contracting for emergency admissions.

We would expect Patients' Charter standards to be reflected in contracts. The Department of Health has just added a new standard for emergency admissions in England: "from April 1995, if you are admitted to hospital through an Accident and Emergency Department, you can expect to be given a bed as soon as possible, and certainly within 3 to 4 hours. From April 1996 this standard will be tightened to 2 hours" The standard in Wales will be two hours from April 1995.

7.1.2   A library of policy documents on emergency services, which have been developed or are being developed in regions and districts, by specialist associations and by Royal Colleges, should be collated by the Health Departments and be accessible to NHS regions, districts and trusts.

We are not aware of a perceived need in the field to support this recommendation. Published documents are available through the normal channels and local documents of possible interest to others may well be brought to wider attention through conferences, meetings etc.

Contracting for urgent and emergency services

7.2.1   Purchasers should contract for and hospitals should receive appropriate funding for the provision of emergency services according to activity and quality in order to balance the present contracting system which tends to encourage elective services.

Purchasers need to purchase the best balance of services to meet the health needs of their population within available resources. Consultant staff can be in a good position to influence contracting decisions using their knowledge of historical patterns of admission and therefore elective bed capacity.

7.2.2   Contracts should provide, to a greater extent than at present, for variations in demand which may arise in time (seasonally or daily in the travelling population) and in place (characteristics of the population and cross boundary flow).

This is a matter for local consideration.

7.2.3   Hospitals' management must give the necessary priority to emergency services.

Hospital managers, in consultation with consultants, are expected to agree with their local purchaser the balance between emergency and elective work.

86

7.2.4   Initiatives such as those to reduce elective waiting lists should be implemented in a way that does not adversely affect the emergency services.

As for 7.2.3.

Admission times

7.3   Health authorities (purchasers) should examine their arrangements and hospitals (providers) should examine their procedures urgently to seek necessary improvements in timing of key events in the admission of urgent or emergency patients.

We agree. Health authorities and hospitals in England were asked in Executive Letter EL(94)8, issued on 20 January 1994, to review the adequacy of their admissions and discharge procedures. That letter also encouraged health authorities to set local Patients' Charter standards for emergency admissions (see 7.1.1 above for the new national standard).

Admission Management

7.4   Hospitals should review the management arrangements for urgent or emergency admission including consideration of the following:

7.4.1   Bed ownership: The move away from traditional "consultant ownership" of beds and towards development of schemes of bed pooling for the appropriate care of urgent and emergency admissions.

7.4.2   Admission wards: The use of admission wards in some form and further operational research into their optimum organisation.

7.4.3   Observation wards in accident and emergency departments: Consideration to the introduction of observation wards and further operational research to identify the best modes of organising them.

7.4.4   Emergency operating theatres: Urgent moves to provide 24 hour availability of emergency theatres.

7.4.5   Bed closures: Collaboration of managers and clinicians to address problems to the emergency services which result from reduced bed capacity when bed closures are necessary.

7.4.6   Bed managers: The appointment of bed managers with appropriate authority and seniority to operate a 24 hour service within agreed protocols.

7.4.7   "Hostel" or "hotel" beds: Operational research to evaluate the role of "hostel" or "hotel" beds and to develop these ideas in the most efficient manner.

7.4.8   Clinical directorates - communication and management: The further development of clinical directorates to ensure the full and continuing collaboration of managers and clinicians in use of resources for emergency services.

7.4.9   Information technology - communications within hospital: Exploitation of potential uses of information technology to facilitate the rapid transfer of relevant information (results of diagnostic tests) and improve communications with consultants on call.

7.4.10   Staffing: Review of nursing and other professional staffing and distribution to meet needs of emergency services.

7.4.11   Availability of support services: Audit of availability and times of obtaining diagnostic and other supporting services to identify shortfalls and delays.

7.4.12   Discharge planning: The appointment of discharge co-ordinators.

This is a useful, though not necessarily exhaustive, checklist of issues which hospitals will wish to consider in the light of local priorities and available resources.

Organisation of services for urgent and emergency admission

7.5.1   Hospital layout and design: When acute care is provided on split- or multiple-sites, consideration should be given to placing all acute specialties on a single site.

This has been seen as desirable for many years and many hospital development projects have the effect of concentrating services in the way suggested.

7.5.2   Consultant-led accident and emergency departments:

7.5.2.1   All accident and emergency departments should be led by a consultant, trained in accident and emergency medicine.

This has been Departmental policy for many years, following the recommendation to this effect in 1971 by a Joint Consultants Committee working group under the Chairmanship of Sir John Bruce. Most accident and emergency departments are consultant led and the majority of such consultants will have been trained specifically in &E medicine; this proportion is likely to increase.

7.5.2.2   Inadequate medical establishment should be resolved by the Health Departments and the Royal Colleges by increasing the number of training posts.

An increase in the number of training posts in A&E was agreed by the Joint Planning Advisory Committee following a review in November 1991.

7.5.2.3   Hand-over arrangements should be agreed so that patients may be admitted without repeated examination by junior trainees (from other departments).

This is for local consideration. All concerned with the patient's management need to be fully aware of the patient's condition and that may lead to unavoidable repeat examinations.

7.5.3   General practitioners:

7.5.3.1   Problems that some general practices have in providing a 24 hour service should be addressed by FHSAs.

We agree. Changes to the ways in which GPs provide emergency medical care for their patients outside surgery hours have recently been agreed with the British Medical Association. These changes reaffirm the GP's 24 hour commitment to his or her patient and the continuing availability of home visits when necessary and appropriate. They also clarify the existing responsibilities of GPs for providing emergency services and open the way for GPs to become better organised in providing care - spending less time on call, but working more intensively, or on a more co-operative basis, when they are on call.

GPs will continue to be responsible for the diagnosis of any illness their patients may have and for arranging appropriate consultation and treatment. In addition, the NHS Executive (in England) is developing a new option for patients who require urgent medical attention out of normal surgery hours: new Primary Care Centres are to be established for diagnosis and treatment.

7.5.3.2   Further studies should be undertaken to address the issue of demand for "primary care" in some accident and emergency departments.

Paragraph 6.21 of the report notes that various methods have been and are being evaluated to alleviate pressures caused by patients seeking "primary care" in accident and emergency departments.

7.5.4   Nurse practitioners: Further evaluation of nurse practitioner schemes in accident and emergency should be undertaken.

We welcome the development of nurse practitioner roles in Accident and Emergency Departments and accept that hospitals may wish to consider producing locally agreed protocols to ensure the nursing care provided suits local circumstances. Nurse practitioner roles are being developed in a wide range of settings. We have already funded a study which examined the prevalence, distribution and scope of nurse practitioners in A&E Departments in England and Wales and last year also assisted financially in the evaluation of nurse practitioner schemes in a variety of community settings in South East Thames Region. In January 1994 we gave £300,000 for ten innovative nurse practitioner projects in acute hospitals and primary care settings.

7.5.5   Psychiatric patients in accident and emergency: Substantive arrangements should be developed in consultation with psychiatrists to deal with problems associated with psychiatric patients in accident and emergency departments.

A number of initiatives are taking place which are examining the range of service provision available for mentally ill people, including the provision of emergency care in accident and emergency departments.

7.5.6   Discharge and social services: solutions should be sought urgently to counter discharge delays attributable to Social Services or Community Care.

7.5.7   "Community care" and services for urgent and emergency admissions: Closer consultation should be developed between separate sectors of health, social and community care to ensure the desirable "seamless" services.

These recommendations are in line with current policy. The new arrangements for community care, which were introduced in April 1993, provide a clear framework for social services and NHS to work together to assess and meet the needs of vulnerable people in the community, including people who are being discharged from hospital. The evidence so far from our monitoring work is that there has been a good start to the new arrangements with few significant problems reported in relation to hospital discharge.

We made this a key priority in local and health authorities' work to prepare for and consolidate the new arrangements. Authorities have been required to produce evidence of agreements on hospital discharge and continuing care responsibilities as a precondition for the Community Care Special Transitional Grant in 1993/4 and 1994/5.

In addition the NHS Executive, Social Services Inspectorate and Audit Commission have recently issued a workbook on hospital discharge to both health and social services staff in England. The workbook provides a self audit and training tool to allow health and social services staff to look at their own performance on hospital discharge and identify areas for improvement. It covers many of the issues raised in the CSAG report. A programme of dissemination workshops for both health and social services staff has been arranged to promote the use of the workbook.

Review of services for urgent and emergency admission

7.6.1   Hospital audit: hospitals should conduct regular audits of issues raised in this report.

We accept that hospital staff will find this a fruitful area for clinical audit.

7.6.2   National review: a further national review of urgent and emergency admissions should be undertaken in two years' time.

We note this recommendation.

January 1995

Printed in the United Kingdom for HMSO.
Dd.0299985, 1/95, C26, 3400, 5673, 303377.